医学机能实验学

（双 语 版，2019）

主编　刘　桦　陈　晨

东南大学出版社

·南京·

图书在版编目(CIP)数据

医学机能实验学:双语版/刘桦,陈晨主编.—南京:东南大学出版社,2019.8(2022.1重印)

ISBN 978-7-5641-5072-3

Ⅰ.①医… Ⅱ.①刘…②陈… Ⅲ.①实验医学—双语教学—高等学校—教材 Ⅳ.①R-33

中国版本图书馆 CIP 数据核字(2014)第 161633 号

出版发行	东南大学出版社
出 版 人	江建中
网　　　址	http://www.seupress.com
电子邮箱	press@seupress.com
社　　　址	南京市四牌楼 2 号
邮　　　编	210096
电　　　话	025-83793191(发行)　025-57711295(传真)
经　　　销	全国各地新华书店
印　　　刷	江苏凤凰数码印务有限公司
开　　　本	787 mm×1092 mm　1/16
印　　　张	8.75
字　　　数	220 千字
版　　　次	2014 年 8 月第 1 版
印　　　次	2022 年 1 月第 3 次印刷
书　　　号	ISBN 978-7-5641-5072-3
定　　　价	28.00 元

本社图书若有印装质量问题,请直接与营销部联系。电话(传真):025-83791830。

《医学机能实验学》(双语版,2019)编委会

主　　编　刘　桦　陈　晨

副 主 编　董　榕　余卫平　吴晓冬　刘莉洁　贺广远

英文审校　王　坚　姚红红

编　　委(按姓氏笔画排序)

王　坚　王晓斌　石丽娟　成于思　朱新建

刘莉洁　刘　桦　寻庆英　孙玲美　吴晓冬

余卫平　沈传陆　杨　健　张　伟　陈　晨

林　琳　易宏伟　赵　蕾　姚红红　贺广远

袁艺标　巢　杰　董　榕　廖　凯　戴小牛

前　　言

现代医学教育以培养医学生综合素质为宗旨,转变教育理念,改革人才培养模式,实现教学内容、课程体系、教学方法和手段的现代化。为了适应创新性人才培养和实验改革的需要,根据生理学、病理生理学和药理学实验教学的共性及现代实验技术发展趋势,将这三门学科的实验教学部分从原课程中分离出来,科学有机地整合成一门新型的综合性和研究性实验课程——医学机能实验学。该实验课程教学作为医学教育的重要组成部分,对培养医学生实践能力、创新意识、科学思维方法和严谨的科学态度至关重要。

医学机能实验课程以活体动物为主要实验对象,以研究机体功能、疾病发生机制和药物作用规律为主要内容。通过机能实验教学,培养学生客观地观察、比较、分析问题的综合能力,培养医学生科学研究的基本素养。

本教材根据教学大纲的要求,结合我校医学院生理学、病理生理学和药理学经典实验教学的特色,由浅入深地进行编排。主要内容包括实验动物的基本概念、常用实验动物技术、实验动物操作的基本规范、多道生物信号采集处理系统原理和其他仪器设备的正确使用、基础性实验、综合性实验、探索性实验、多媒体虚拟实验、病案讨论、实验设计等。为配合我院全英文教学以及来华留学生教学需要,实验部分采用中、英两种文字编写,便于读者对照阅读。

本次教材修订是由长期从事机能实验教学的诸位老师与机能实验中心技术人员积极合作共同完成,承蒙东南大学医学院的大力支持,在此表示衷心感谢。由于条件所限,欠缺或不妥之处难免。在此,恳请广大师生提出宝贵意见,使之不断完善。

编　者

2019 年 6 月

目　　录

第一章 绪 论

第一节 机能实验学的性质和任务

机能实验学是一门以活体实验动物为主要研究对象,以探讨机体正常生理功能、疾病发生机制和药物作用规律为主要内容的实验学科,是生理学、病理生理学、药理学3门学科实验内容有机融合的一门综合性实验学科。目前该实验课程内容主要包括两个方面:一是主要在整体和器官水平上观察机体功能和代谢的变化规律,包括正常生理功能变化、疾病过程中和药物作用下对机体功能和代谢的影响;二是将生理学、病理生理学、药理学3门学科实验内容进行了有机整合,由单一学科实验内容到3门学科的综合实验,并充分运用现代教育技术,比较系统全面地学习和掌握各种实验动物知识和操作技能,提高学生对探索未知问题的兴趣。

通过本课程的学习,学生可以学习到机能实验学的基本方法和常用仪器装置,掌握机能实验学的基本技能和基本操作,认识人体及其他生物体的正常功能、疾病模型及药物作用的基本规律,培养学生科学研究的基本素质,培养学生对事物进行客观观察、比较、分析和综合的能力,以及独立思考、解决实际问题的能力。机能实验教学作为医学教育的重要组成部分,对培养医学生实践能力、创新意识、科学思维方法和严谨的科学态度至关重要。

第二节 机能实验学的教学目的和基本要求

一、机能实验学的教学目的

本课程旨在通过实验教学训练医学生基本操作技能,培养其动手能力。将3门学科的理论知识融会贯通,培养学生实事求是、严谨的科学作风,严密的科学逻辑思维方法,以及观察、分析解决问题的综合能力。通过机能实验基本操作,提高学生的实践动手能力。熟悉机能学实验的基本方法和常用仪器设备的使用。综合运用生理学、病理生理学和药理学等学科的理论知识和实验方法,初步建立整体、全面、系统的疾病观。认识机体的正常功能代谢、疾病模型复制、药物作用基本规律及常用研究方法。通过实验设计,培养学生对实验研究的兴趣,激发学生的创新意识及科学的思维能力,提高综合分析问题和解决问题的能力,养成理论联系实际,勇于探索的科学精神以及团体协作精神。通过病案讨论,培养学生分析病例的能力和对所学知识的综合运用能力,为临床实践打下坚实的基础。通过实验报告的书写和科研论文的撰写,提高学生写作科研论文的能力。

二、机能实验学的教学要求

（一）实验前

（1）预习实验教材，了解每一次实验目的、要求、操作步骤和方法。

（2）结合实验内容，复习实验相关理论知识，理解实验设计的基本原理，预测实验中可能出现的问题，做到心中有数，避免实验中出现不必要的差错和忙乱。

（3）检查领到的器材是否齐全，如果有缺失或者损坏，及时向老师报告。

（二）实验中

（1）遵守实验室规章制度，保持安静和良好的课堂秩序，不做与实验无关的事，尊重老师指导。

（2）实验器材摆放整齐，按照操作规程正确使用仪器和手术器械。公用试剂和仪器不得随意移动位置，以免影响他人使用。

（3）保护实验动物和标本，节约试剂和药品，爱护实验器材、实验仪器或器械，切忌违规操作或粗暴使用。如在实验过程中意外损坏实验器械，应向老师报告说明，以便及时检修或更换。故意损坏实验仪器或器械者，除照价赔偿外，学校将给予处罚。

（4）计算机操作时应掌握如何正确开机、如何进入实验程序、如何启动记录、如何存储与输出、如何打印实验结果及关机等。严禁在计算机上玩游戏、新建个人文件、随意启动其他程序，甚至损坏实验程序以及与实验无关（甚至非法）的活动。

（5）各实验小组既要分工负责，又要团结协作，按照实验步骤，以严肃认真的态度操作。实验过程要胆大心细，操作规范，认真记录实验中的现象，实事求是记录实验结果。实验过程中，应仔细耐心地观察并记录每项实验出现的结果。实验记录要做到客观、具体、清楚、完整。

（6）认真仔细地观察实验中出现的现象，积极主动思考和分析实验结果和现象，力求理解每个实验步骤和实验结果的意义。

（三）实验后

（1）关闭电源，整理实验仪器及桌面物品。

（2）洗净手术器械并摆放整齐，如数归还。能重复利用的器材（如纱布、缝合针、试管、插管、针头等）应洗净再用。

（3）按照规定妥善处理实验后的废物和动物标本。实验废物不得乱倒、乱扔，尤其是强酸、强碱试剂，动物被毛、组织器官、纸屑等不得倒入水槽内，应统一放置在指定地点。

（4）值日生做好实验室的清洁卫生，打扫地面卫生，关好门窗水电。最后，请实验室管理人员检查验收后方能离开。

（5）整理实验数据，对实验结果进行分析讨论，认真书写实验报告并按时交给老师评阅。

第三节　实验结果的记录方法和实验报告书写要求

一、实验结果的记录方法

对于实验结果的表述，一般有以下 3 种方法：

（1）文字叙述：根据实验目的将原始资料系统化、条理化，尽量用准确的医学术语客观地描述实验现象和结果。

（2）图表形式：用表格或坐标图方式总结实验结果，便于相互比较，尤其适合于分组较多，且各组观察指标一致的实验。每一图表应有表题和计量单位。

（3）曲线图：用记录仪器（如 RM6240 EC 多道生理信号采集系统）描记出的曲线图，指标的变化趋势更加直观（如血压、呼吸曲线和心电图等），变化趋势通过曲线图直观明了。在实验报告中，可任选其中一种或几种方法并用，以获得最佳效果。

二、实验报告的书写要求

实验报告是机能实验学的重要组成部分，是从感性认识到理性认识的升华过程，是以实验结果为依据的科学推理分析过程，是提高学生科研能力的一条重要途径，所以实验课要求学生一定要撰写实验报告。实验报告的内容一般格式包括：

（1）实验名称：概括实验的主要内容。一般将实验题目放在实验报告纸的第一行靠左或居中。

（2）实验目的及原理：反映本次实验的主要意义。字数不宜繁多，一般用一两句话阐明实验所要证实的论点或要研究的内容和基本原理即可。

（3）实验器材：要求列出实验所用主要器材。

（4）试剂及药品：要求列出实验所用主要试剂及药品。

（5）实验对象：所用实验动物，数量以及规格。

（6）实验方法与步骤：简明扼要拟出主要操作要点。

（7）实验结果：应将实验过程中观察到的结果实事求是地记录并表述清楚。

（8）讨论和结论：讨论应结合实验结果进行，宜简明扼要。讨论主要是分析、解释所观察到的实验结果和现象。如为预期结果，应结合理论知识对其作用、作用机制进行阐述；如未达预期结果，应找出原因，总结其经验教训。结论放在实验讨论后，作为结尾完成。结论应以实验结果为依据，在讨论的基础上概括并总结出具有代表性的实验结果的论点或推论。可依次概括为：总结结果、寻找规律、推理分析、导出观点、得出结论。

第四节　机能实验室守则

（1）严格考勤制度，按时上下课，认真做好每一项实验。

（2）实验中要听从指导教师的指导，严格遵守各项操作规程。

（3）爱护仪器设备，操作之前必须了解仪器的工作原理和操作程序，不经指导教师批准，不准自行接通或断开电源。

（4）要爱护一切设施，节约实验原材，爱护实验动物。

（5）用酒精灯或易燃物品时，要严防发生火灾。

（6）如发生被实验动物咬伤抓伤等意外情况，应立即报告、及时处理。

（7）实验室应保持安静和整洁，不准随地吐痰、吸烟、吃东西、喧哗和打闹。

（8）实验课结束后，检查仪器，实验器材清洗摆放整齐后归还到实验准备室。

（9）值日生在全部实验结束后搞好实验室卫生，关好门窗水电。

（刘桦　陈晨）

第二章 机能实验学基础

第一节 实验动物科学的概念及研究内容

一、实验动物科学的概念

实验动物科学(laboratory animal science)是研究实验动物和动物实验的一门新兴学科。前者是以实验动物本身为对象,专门研究其育种、繁殖生产、饲养管理、质量监测、疾病诊治和预防以及支撑条件的建立等,即如何培育出标准化的实验动物;后者以实验动物为材料,采用各种手段和方法在实验动物身上进行实验,研究实验过程中实验动物的反应、表现及其发生机制和发展规律,确保动物实验的可靠性、准确性和可重复性,即如何使动物试验合理化、规范化。简而言之,实验动物科学就是关于实验动物标准化和动物实验规范化的科学。

二、实验动物科学研究的范围

(一)实验动物科学研究的内容

实验动物科学,自1950年代诞生以来,至今已成为一门具有自己理论体系的独立性学科,它的主要内容包括:实验动物饲养学、实验动物医学、比较医学、动物实验技术。

(1)实验动物饲养学(laboratory animal breeding science)主要研究实验动物的生物学特性与解剖生理特点、饲育与管理、育种与繁殖、生长与发育、饲料与营养、环境与设施、生态与行为等内容以及实验动物标准化的各种技术、手段和措施。

(2)实验动物医学(laboratory animal medicine)研究实验动物各种疾病包括传染性疾病、营养代谢性疾病、遗传性疾病以及劣质环境所致的疾病的病因、症状、病理特征,疾病的发生、发展规律、诊断、防治措施等;研究实验动物微生物质量的等级标准、检测方法、控制措施以及微生物对动物实验的干扰;研究人畜共患病的预防、控制与治疗措施等。

(3)比较医学(comparative medicine)以实验动物为替身研究人类、造福人类。通过建立人类疾病的动物模型,进行人与动物的类比研究,探讨人类疾病的病因、发生发展规律、预防控制及治疗措施,最终战胜人类的疾病。比较医学又可分成比较解剖学、比较生理学、比较病理学、比较外科学和比较基因组学等。

(4)动物实验技术(animal experiment technique)是进行动物实验时的各种实验手段、技术、方法和标准化操作程序,即在实验室内人为地改变环境条件,观察并记录动物的反应与变化,以探讨生命科学中的疑难问题,获得新的认识,探索新的规律。同时也探讨实验动物科学中的减少、替代、优化问题。

（二）实验动物科学所涉及的领域

1．生命科学领域

生命科学的研究离不开应用实验动物。在对人的各种生理、病理现象和机制以及疾病的防治等研究中，实验动物是人的替难者。譬如，癌症是威胁人类健康的最大疾病，由于在肿瘤的移植、免疫、治疗等研究中使用了裸鼠、悉生动物和无菌动物，人们对各种恶性肿瘤的致癌原因，尤其是化学致癌物质、病毒致癌、肿瘤的病毒、免疫、治疗等方面和研究有了极大的进展，计划生育研究也有相当大的工作是在动物身上做的。各种疾病如高血压、动脉硬化、心脏病、糖尿病、肥胖症、肺炎、神经系统疾病、精神病、胃病、肾病、肺病等的发病、治疗与痊愈的机制及其生理、生化、病理、免疫等各方面的机理，都经过动物实验加以阐明或证实。可以说离开了实验动物和动物实验生命科学就寸步难行。

2．制药工业和化学工业领域

制药和化学工业对实验动物的依赖更为明显。药物和化工产品的副作用，对生命的影响程度包括致癌、致病、致畸、致毒、致突变、致残、致命，都是从实验动物的试验中获得结果。制药和化学工业产品如不用实验动物进行安全评价，包括"三致"（致癌、致畸、致突变）试验，给人类应用将会造成十分严重的恶果。

3．畜牧科学方面

疫苗的制备和鉴定、生理试验、胚胎学研究、营养价值的评估、保持健康群体以及淘汰污染动物等工作，都要使用实验动物。特别是在畜禽传染病的研究工作中，常急需要有合格的实验动物进行实验。

4．农业科学方面

新的优良品种的确立除要做物理的、化学的分析以外，利用实验动物进行生物学的鉴定是十分重要和有意义的。化学肥料、农药的残毒检测，粮食、经济作物品质的优劣等，最后也还是要通过利用实验动物的试验来确定。

5．轻工业科学方面

人们的吃穿用，包括食品、食品添加剂、皮毛及化学纤维、生活日常用品，特别是化学制品有害成份的影响，都要用实验动物去试验。

6．重工业和环境保护方面

在重工业上，对有害物的鉴定和防治，以及国土的整个环境保护，包括废弃物、气体、光辐射、声干扰等各方面的研究工业中，实验动物都是监测的前哨和研究防治措施的标样。

7．国防和军事科学方面

各种武器杀伤效果，化学、辐射、细菌、激光武器的效果和防护，以及在宇宙、航天科学试验中，实验动物都作为人类的替身而取得有价值的科学数据。

8．商品鉴定和国际贸易方面

在进出口商品的检验检疫中，许多商品的质量检验都规定必须进行动物实验鉴定，或直接利用警犬、警鼠担任安全警察，它直接影响着对外贸易的数量、质量和信誉。

9．行为科学的研究方面

实验动物在行为科学的研究中也占有重要地位。例如，汽车设计中的碰撞击实验、土建设计中震动的允许程度、灾难性事故的处理等，国外已经采用实验动物模拟人类的承受极限。

10. 实验动物科学本身研究方面

在实验动物科学本身研究中,由于其综合性很强,涉及数学、物理、化学、生物学、动物学、胚胎学、营养学、微生物学、遗传学、解剖组织学、寄生虫学、传染病学、免疫学、血液学、麻醉学、生态学、建筑学等,所以,各个学科与实验动物科学相辅相成,相互渗透。虽然它的直接研究目的是取得适用于各种特性需要的实验动物,但对生命科学的微观领域,都进行了更为深入的探索,例如,在遗传学、生殖生理学等的科学以及实用技术方面,都不断取得突破。

实验动物科学应用如此广泛,主要是由实验动物的特点所决定的。实验动物具有无菌或已知菌丛、遗传背景明确、模型性状显著且稳定、纯度高、敏感性强、反应性一致、重现性好以及繁殖快(世代间隔短)、产仔多、价格相对低廉等特点。可以满足各种不同研究要求和生产需要,因而广泛应用于医学、兽医学、药学、营养学、农学、畜牧学、劳动保护、环境保护、计划生育与优生、食品与饮料添加物、日用化妆品、化纤织物以及生命科学等领域。

三、医学与实验动物科学

(一) 医学研究离不开实验动物

据有关资料统计,生物学和医学实验中 60% 的课题要用到实验动物。

医学科学的使命是消除人类的一切疾病,保证健康,延年益寿。而它所面临的生命现象是自然界中各种现象中最复杂的一种,经过了漫长的进化,生命现象呈现出难以设想的精微、细密、巧妙与和谐,要研究其中无限纷繁、盘根错节、众多方面的因果联系,进一步掌握其本质和规律,实非易事,可以想见,对人体本身的观察分析和认识,是有限制的,不方便的。以人为对象进行研究,所得到的材料是宝贵的,其结论可直接有益于人。但是,这种研究非常困难,不少观测和研究,根本不可能进行。以人为对象进行研究,无论是在方法上、条件上,还是在处置上,结论上都有很多限制或困难,势必造成医学发展迟缓,不利于防治人类的疾病和维护人体的健康。因此,离开动物实验,很难设想医学的进步!

然而,人的认识能力的发展是无止境的,人们在医学研究中采用生物学的,化学的,物理学的以至数学的方法进行各种医学问题的实验探索和观测,阐明生命活动在正常条件和异常条件下的表现与规律,了解它、控制它、利用它或改变它。更为可贵的是研究者们成功地找到"替代者"——实验动物。用实验动物来进行研究,就不再受方法上、手段上、条件上、时间上的限制了,基于伦理道德考虑的限制因素也减少了,可以进行前瞻性研究(即预先设计),可以进行验证,可以反复地试验,可以随时获取各种活体标本。

巴甫洛夫曾指出:"没有对活的动物进行的实验和观察,人们就无法认识有机界的各种规律,这是无可争辩的"。

(二) 实验动物科技进步促进医学的发展

从活体解剖动物到现代解剖学基础,从动物血液循环到现代生理学的建立,从"神农尝百草"到现代药理学、毒理学的发展,从传染病病原的发现到现代免疫学的创立,从物种起源到细胞的发现再到 DNA 双螺旋结构的阐明,每一个新的领域,每一个新的发现,每一个重大进展,无一不是通过动物实验来实现的。

临床医学的许多重大技术的创新和发展也与动物实验紧密相连。新的手术方法、麻醉方法的确立,体外循环、心脏外科、断肢再植、器官或组织移植、肿瘤的切除与治疗等各项工作的开展也无一不是在动物实验的基础上发展起来的。离开了实验动物科学,医学的进步与发展只能是一句空话。

由于研究的需要，人们培育出了近交系动物、突变系动物、杂交一代动物；转基因动物、基因敲除动物、克隆动物也应运而生。由于研究的需要，人们饲育出了无特定病原体动物、无菌动物。由于培育、饲养各种特殊实验动物的需要，人们发明了特殊的育种、保种技术，建立了专门的饲养、繁殖技术。科学家们把现代光学技术、电子技术、显微摄影及成像技术应用于实验动物科学研究，把环境控制、空气净化、自动控制、建筑工程等工程技术运用到实验动物和动物实验设施的建立，把现代信息技术运用于实验动物管理，促进了实验动物的标准化和动物实验的规范化。从而使得各国科学家的有关研究能够取得可靠的结果和良好的反应重复性，开展国际合作，进行国际交流。

现代分子生物学技术加快了实验动物新品系的培育速度，建立各种人类疾病动物模型有了更好的手段和更广阔的空间。反过来，新的品系和动物模型的建立又为医学、药学、遗传学等生命科学的各个领域提供了可靠而有用的手段和先进的工具。

生物大分子结构是体现其功能的基础，不仅生物大分子的一级结构变异可引起疾病（称作分子病），二级结构和高级结构的改变也可引起疾病，如"构象病""离子通道病""受体病""细胞骨架病""分子伴侣病""信号传导病"等，不一而足，这些"结构病"实质为"功能病"，因而结构与功能的关系成为分子生物学所致力探讨的主题之一。由于基因的碱基序列、转录和翻译、蛋白质的加工、修饰和剪接等都可使生命功能多样化，决定功能表现的遗传学背景、遗传信息的传递过程、分子间的相互作用和调控，必须综合起来去考虑，才能找出发病原因和机制，并找到诊断、治疗和预防的办法。而这种研究离开了实验动物科学的平台，就只能停留于结构研究，难以深入其功能研究。

（三）实验动物质量与医学研究的关系

在生命科学研究领域内，进行实验研究所需要的基本条件可以总括为实验动物、设备、信息和试剂，称为生命科学研究四要素，简称 AEIR 四要素。这 4 个要素，在整个实验研究中，具有同等重要的地位，不能忽略或偏废。事实上，实验动物质量往往成为制约性要素，影响整个实验的质量和水平。

保持实验动物质量标准必须实行实验动物微生物学及遗传学的严格质量控制，排除所有可能影响动物质量、干扰实验结果、甚至有可能危害人的健康的细菌、病毒和寄生虫；饲养和使用遗传背景明确、可控、通用的的品系动物，是动物实验取得成功的前提条件。

在实践中，往往有些研究人员对实验动物的质量标准不够重视，认为动物是活的就能用；或者是只关注了实验动物的质量，而忽视了实验环境的质量，将高等级的实验动物拿到一般环境中做实验。更有甚者，将实验后的观察动物饲养于严重不合规定的恶劣环境中，与实验动物福利的原则相背离。也有的研究者，既有高质量的实验动物，也有标准化的实验环境和条件，但不会使用，不按规范使用，不执行管理条例，浪费资源，违背科学，违反法规。诸如此类，累见不鲜，结果导致实验的失败；或即使完成了实验，其实验结果令人怀疑，成果得不到科技主管部门的认可，更难得到国外同行的承认。当然，由于认识上的差距，有些人舍得花钱买仪器设备和试剂，却不舍得花钱饲养或购买实验动物，殊不知，实验动物是医学研究关键性的限制性要素，直接影响着科研水平的高低。

实验动物生产条件与动物实验条件必须按照国际标准严格控制，并尽可能一致，才能保持实验动物质量的一致性和可靠性，才不会造成高等级实验动物进入低等级实验环境中而导致实验动物质量降级或降质。同时也应防止低等级动物进入高等级设施而污染整个环境。

医学研究的最终结果都要应用于人类,与人类的健康息息相关。因此,来不得半点马虎,所有研究者都必须高度重视实验动物的质量问题。

四、实验动物科学发展趋势

(一)重视动物福利

1. 动物保护

动物保护是人类对赖以生存的环境及自身命运进行深层次的思考之后提出的一个重要课题。伴随着经济的发展和社会的进步,动物保护的观念在人们的思想和生活中得以体现。它是保护生物多样性、环境生态平衡以及人类生存和发展的需要,是社会进步的表现。动物保护主要包括两个方面的内容:一是对濒危动物物种和种群的保存,以维持生态平衡;二是对动物个体生命的保护和保健,使动物免受伤害或疾病的折磨。不同的人群,关注不同的动物群体,我们所关注的是为科研目的而驯化、饲养的实验动物。

从实验动物科学的层面上讲,动物保护的最好做法是善待动物,给动物以好的生活、生存条件,保证动物的健康。尽可能少地、科学合理地使用实验动物,规范地开展各种动物实验。同时,开展各种替代方法的研究。

2. 动物福利

动物福利是动物在整个生命过程中动物保护的具体体现,其基本原则是保证动物的康乐(well-being)。动物康乐包括使动物身体健康,体质健壮,行为正常,无心理的紧张、压抑和痛苦等。从理论上讲,动物康乐的标准是对动物需求的满足。动物的需求包括三个方面,即维持生命的需要、维持健康的需要以及生活舒适的需要。动物福利的目的是为了动物的康乐,是保证动物康乐的外部条件,而动物康乐的状态又反映了动物福利条件的状况。搞好动物福利的前提是提高对动物福利的认识,从各个环节去保证为动物创造符合动物要求的生存、居住、生活条件,维护动物的健康;对研究人员来说,还必须考虑通过优化设计,减少实验动物的用量,减轻动物的不安和疼痛,给予良好的术后护理,实验结束或实验过程中获取标本应采取安乐死的方法等。

搞好实验动物福利的直接受益者是实验者,能够确保实验动物质量,确保实验结果的准确、可靠、可比、科学有效。而最终真正的受益者是整个人类。

(二)减少、替代和优化研究不断深化和发展

在西方国家动物是人的朋友,用动物做实验常受到各种指责和非议。我国已加入了WTO,要顺应世界潮流,开拓国际市场,我国的实验动物工作者和各级领导必须认真研究、高度重视西方国家的动物保护组织和动物保护运动。当前在西方国家受动物保护运动的影响,在实验动物行业内,兴起了"3R"运动,即动物实验的减少、替代和优化。

减少(reduction):选用恰当的高质量的实验动物进行动物实验,改进实验设计,提高实验动物的利用率,从而减少动物的使用数量。

替代(replacement):以低等生物、微生物或细胞、组织、器官甚至电子计算机模拟、替代活动物实验。采用替代的方法必须经过反复的验证,在保证实验结果科学、可靠、可比较的前提下,来替代动物实验。

优化(refinement):主要指实验技术路线和手段的精细设计和选择,减少实验动物的紧

张与不适,减轻动物的痛苦,使动物实验有更好的结果,保证动物实验的可重复性。

"3R"运动最终使实验动物的使用量逐步减少,质量要求愈来愈高,动物实验结果的准确性、可靠性也不断提高。"3R"反映了实验动物科学由技术上的严格要求转向人道主义的管理,提倡实验动物福利与动物保护的国际总趋势。

(三) 实验动物标准化,资源多样化

实验动物标准化由实验动物生产条件的标准化、实验动物质量的标准化、动物实验条件的标准化以及与之相适应的饲养管理规范化和动物实验规范化几个部分组成。只有具备了标准化的生产条件,严格执行饲养管理标准操作规程,才能生产出标准化的实验动物;只有具备了标准化的实验动物和标准化的动物实验条件,执行标准实验操作规程,才有可能得出可靠的实验结果;只有实验结果准确、可靠、可重复,实验研究才有价值、有意义。

现代科学的发展要求应用更多种类、品系、高质量的实验动物以及各种疾病动物模型,作为应用学科的实验动物学必然以科学的需求为自身的发展方向。目前,已开展了许多种类的动物,如沙鼠、白化高原鼠兔、小型猪、树鼩、土拔鼠、非人灵长类等野生哺乳动物的实验动物化研究;水生动物如剑尾鱼、斑马鱼、红鲫的实验动物化研究等等。

对现有实验动物通过各种技术手段包括分子生物学的手段、化学或物理诱变的手段、胚胎操作技术、特殊的育种手段等,培育各种有用的动物模型供科学研究使用,具有非常好的发展前景。基因治疗药物的研制,生物反应器的研制与开发,各种新的疾病如 SARS 的治疗与预防都有赖于新的动物模型的开发。因此,实验动物资源多样性是必然趋势。

(四) 动物实验规范化

要保证动物实验取得准确、可靠、可信、可重复的结果,必须规范动物实验,只有规范的动物实验才有可比性。要规范动物实验,就必须实施优良实验室操作规范(good laboratory practice,GLP)。各国的 GLP 规范其基本原则一致、内容也基本相同。因此,经 GLP 认证的实验室,能够得到国际承认。一个与国际接轨的动物实验室,同样应通过 GLP 验收。概括起来,GLP 规范主要包括实验室人员的组成和职责,设施、设备运行维护和环境控制,动物品系、级别和质量控制标准,质量保证部门、标准操作规程(SOP)、受试品和对照品的接受与管理、非临床实验室研究的实验方案、实验记录和总结报告等。GLP 实验室的正常运行,人员素质是关键,实验设施是基础,SOP 是手段,质量监督是保证,硬件是外壳,软件是核心。只有推进 GLP 规范,才能做到动物实验的规范化。

(王晓斌)

第二节　常用实验动物的基本操作技术

一、常用实验动物的生物学特征

1. 蛙(或蟾蜍)

蛙(蟾蜍)属于两栖变温动物,皮肤光滑湿润,有腺体、无外鳞。蛙的心脏有 2 个心房,1 个心室,心房与心室区分不明显,动静脉血液混合,有冬眠习性。生存环境比哺乳动物简单,在机能学实验中有多种实验选择该类动物。如:①离体蛙心实验,常用来研究心脏的生理功

能及药物对心脏活动的影响；②蛙的腓肠肌和坐骨神经可用于观察外周神经及其肌肉的功能，以及药物对周围神经、骨骼肌或神经肌肉接头的影响；③缝匠肌可用于记录终板电位、脊休克、脊髓反射、反射弧分析、肠系膜微循环等。

2. 小白鼠

小白鼠性情温顺，易于捕捉，胆小怕惊，对外来刺激敏感。它胃容量小，不耐饥渴，随时采食，易饲养，故适用于需求量大的实验动物。在机能学实验中常选用该动物，如：某些药物的筛选实验、半数致死量（LD50）测定、药效比较、毒性实验、避孕药实验及抗癌药实验。

3. 大白鼠

大白鼠性情温顺，行动迟缓，易于捕捉，但受惊吓或粗暴操作时，会紧张不安甚至攻击人。大鼠嗅觉发达，对外界刺激敏感，抵抗力较强。大鼠无胆囊，肾单位表浅，肝再生能力强。大鼠的血压反应比兔稳定，可用它作血压实验，也可用于慢性实验、抗炎、降脂、利胆、子宫实验及心血管系统的实验。药典规定该动物为催产素效价测定及药品指控中升压物质检查指定动物。

4. 豚鼠

豚鼠性情温和，胆小，饲养管理方便，可群养。豚鼠耳蜗管发达，听觉灵敏，存在可见的普赖厄反射（听觉耳动反射），乳突部骨质薄弱。豚鼠对组织胺、人型结核杆菌很敏感。其自身不能制造维生素 C，是研究实验性坏血症的唯一动物。

5. 家兔

家兔属于草食性动物，性情温顺但群居性差，听觉、嗅觉十分灵敏，胆小易惊，具夜行性和嗜睡性。它主要利用呼吸散热维持体温平衡，耐冷不耐热，厌湿喜干。家兔广泛应用于医学研究中。由于兔耳血管丰富，耳静脉表浅，易暴露，是静脉给药及采血的最佳部位。兔的减压神经在颈部与迷走交感神经分开走行而自成一束，常用于研究减压神经与心血管活动的关系。家兔的体温调节较稳定，反应灵敏，常用于发热研究和热源试验，是药品质控中热源检查的指定动物。家兔对组织胺不敏感，不发生呕吐，因此不适用于组织胺过敏性休克、催吐和镇吐药物的研究。

6. 狗

狗品种繁多，个体差异大。听、嗅觉灵敏，反应敏捷，对外界环境适应能力强，易驯养，经过训练后能很好地配合实验。狗在基础医学研究和教学实验中是最常用的实验动物之一。常用于心血管系统、脊髓传导、大脑皮层功能定位、条件反射、内分泌腺摘除和各种消化系统功能的实验研究。特别适用于实验外科学的研究，是临床探索新的手术方法和观察手术疗效的首选实验动物。

二、常见实验动物的捉持和给药方法

1. 蛙（或蟾蜍）捉持和给药方法

（1）捉持方法

通常以左手握持，用食指和中指夹住左前肢，拇指压住右前肢，右手将下肢拉直，用左手无名指及小指夹住（图 2-1）。

（2）给药方法

一般将药物注射于胸、腹或股淋巴囊。因其皮肤较薄，为避免药液从针眼中漏出，故作胸部淋巴囊注射时，针头由口腔

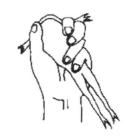

图 2-1　蟾蜍捉持方法

底部穿下颌肌层而达胸部皮下;作股部淋巴囊注射时,应从小腿皮肤刺入,通过膝关节而达大腿部皮下。注入药量一般为 0.25～0.5 ml。

2. 小白鼠的捉持和给药方法

(1) 捉持方法

右手提起鼠尾,放在粗糙物(如鼠笼)上面,轻向后拉其尾;此时小鼠前肢抓住粗糙面不动;用左手拇指和食指捏住双耳及头部皮肤,无名指、小指和掌心夹其背部皮肤及尾部,便可将小鼠完全固定(图 2-2)。腾出右手,可以给药。

此外,也可单手捉持,难度较大,但速度快。先用拇指和食指抓住小鼠尾巴,用小指、无名指和手掌压住尾根部,再用腾出的拇指、食指及中指抓住鼠双耳及头部皮肤而固定。

(2) 给药方法

① 灌胃法:小鼠固定后,使腹部朝上,颈部拉直,右手用带灌胃针头的注射器吸取药液(或事先将药液吸好),将针头从口角插入口腔,再从舌背进沿上腭进入食道(图 2-3)。若遇阻力,应退出后再插,切不可用力过猛,防止损伤或误入气管导致动物死亡。灌胃量一般不超过 0.25 ml/10 g 体重。

② 腹腔注射:抓鼠方法同上,右手持注射器(5～6 号针头),从耻骨联合上一侧向头端以 45° 角刺入腹腔(应避开膀胱)(图 2-4)。可先刺入皮下 2～3 mm,再刺入腹腔,以防药液外漏。针头刺入部位不宜太高太深,以免刺破内脏。注射量一般为 0.1～0.25 ml/10 g 体重。

③ 皮下注射法:一般两人合作。一人左手抓住小鼠头部皮肤,右手拉住鼠尾;另一人左手提高背部皮肤,右手持住注射器(针头号同上),将针头刺入提起的皮下(图 2-5)。若一人操作,左手小指和手掌夹住鼠尾,拇指和食指提起背部皮肤,右手持注射器给药。一般用量不超过 0.25 ml/10 g 体重。

④ 肌肉注射法:两人合作时,一人抓鼠方法同图 2-5,另一人左手拉直一侧后肢,右手持注射器,注射部位多选后腿上部外侧(针头号同上)。如一人操作,抓鼠方法类似腹腔注射,只是药液注射在肌肉内。每条腿的注射量不宜超过 0.1 ml/10 g 体重。

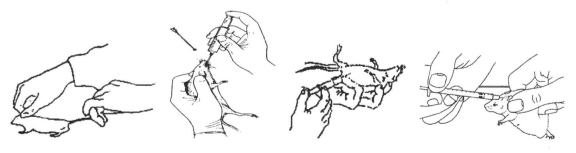

图 2-2 小鼠固定　　　图 2-3 小鼠灌胃　　　图 2-4 腹腔注射　　　图 2-5 皮下注射

⑤ 尾静脉注射法:将小鼠置于待置的固定筒内,使鼠尾外露,并用酒精或二甲苯棉球涂擦,或插入 40～50℃ 温水中浸泡片刻,使尾部血管扩张。左手拉尾,选择扩张最明显的血管;右手持注射器(4～5 号针头),将针头刺入血管,缓慢给药。如推注有阻力而且局部变白,说明针头不在血管内,应重新穿刺。穿刺时宜从近尾尖部 1/3 处静脉开始,以便重复

向上移位注射（图 2-6）。一般用药量为 0.1～0.2 ml/10 g 体重，不宜超过 0.5 ml/10 g 体重。

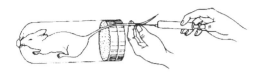

图 2-6　尾静脉注射

3. 大白鼠的捉持和给药方法

（1）捉持方法

大白鼠比小白鼠攻击性强，捉持前先戴上手套，右手夹住尾巴，放在粗糙面上；左手拇指和食指捏住颈及前颈部，其余三指握住整个身体。用力适当，过松容易挣脱而被咬伤，但用力过大会使其窒息死亡。

（2）给药方法

类似于小白鼠，只是用药量加大一些，静脉给药除尾静脉注射外还可舌下静脉给药。

4. 豚鼠的捉持和给药方法

（1）捉持方法

豚鼠性情温和，可直接用左手抓住身体即可，或以左手抓住其头颈部，右手抓住两后肢。

（2）给药方法

皮下、肌肉及腹腔注射方法与小白鼠类似，只是用药量稍大。灌胃方法与兔类似（见后述）。静脉注射方法，可选后脚掌外侧静脉、外颈部静脉、或作股静脉切开注射。作后脚掌外侧静脉注射时，有一人提豚鼠并固定一条后腿，另一人剪去注射部位的毛，用酒精棉球涂擦后脚掌外侧的皮肤，使血管显露。再将连在注射器上的小儿头皮静脉输液针头刺入血管。作外颈静脉注射时需先剪去一点皮肤，使血管暴露，然后将针头刺入。豚鼠的静脉管壁比较脆弱，操作时需特别小心。

5. 家兔的捉持和给药方法

（1）捉持方法

一般左手抓住兔颈背部皮肤，将其提起，右手托住臀部呈坐姿（图 2-7）。不要抓两耳，以防兔挣扎。

（2）给药方法

① 耳缘静脉注射法：一人操作时，将兔放入固定箱或试验台上，选好耳缘静脉（在耳背的下缘），拔除局部的毛，用酒精棉球涂擦，并用食指轻弹耳壳，使血管扩张。用左手的食指和中指夹住耳根部，拇指和无名指夹住耳尖部拉直；右手将抽好药液的注射器（6～7 号针头）刺入血管，用拇指和食指使针头和兔耳固定，将药液推入（图 2-8）。如针头在血管内，推注轻松，并可见血液被药液冲

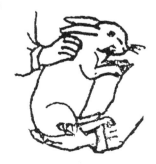

图 2-7　家兔捉持

走；如不在血管内，则推注有阻力，耳局部变白或肿胀，应立即拔除重新注射。注射完毕，则用手指或棉球压在针眼上，再拔出针头，并继续按压片刻，防止出血。如两人操作，一人捉住兔子，右手暴露血管，压住耳根部使血管充盈，另一人注射给药。一般用药量为 0.2～2.0 ml/kg 体重。

② 灌胃法：两人合作，一人坐下，两腿夹住兔身，左手固定兔耳，右手抓住前肢；另一人将开口器从嘴角插入口腔，压在舌上，并向后翻转几下，使兔舌伸直。取 8 号导尿管由开口器中部的小孔插入食道约 15 cm（图 2-9）。如插入气管，兔子则剧烈挣扎、呼吸困难。也可

将导尿管外端浸入水中,不见气泡则表示插在胃中。插好后,把注射器接在导尿管上,将药液推入。再注入少量空气,使导尿管中所有药液进入胃内。灌完药液后,先慢慢抽出导尿管,再取出开口器。一般用药量为 5～20 ml/kg 体重。

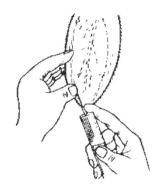

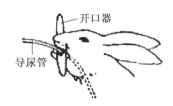

图 2-8　兔耳缘静脉注射　　　　　　图 2-9　兔灌胃

6. 狗

(1) 捉持方法

驯服的狗可戴上特制嘴套,用绳带固定于耳后颈部;凶暴的狗可用长柄捕狗夹钳住狗的颈部,然后套上嘴套。狗嘴也可用绳带固定,操作时先将绳带绕过狗嘴的下颌打结,再绕到颈后部打结,以防绳带滑落。狗麻醉后四肢固定于手术台上,取下嘴套或绳带,将一金属棒经两侧嘴角,穿过口腔压于舌上,再用绳带绕过金属棒绑缚狗嘴,并固定于手术台上。应将狗舌拉出口腔,以防窒息。

(2) 给药方法

① 静脉注射法:可选用前肢皮下大静脉或后肢小隐静脉注射。以手或橡皮带把静脉向心端扎紧,使血管充血。酒精棉球涂檫后,针头向近心端刺入静脉,回抽针栓,若有回血即可推注药液(图2-10-a)。

② 肌肉注射法:选择两侧臀部或股部肌肉。在固定动物后,注射器与肌肉成 60°,一次刺入肌肉注射,但应避免针刺入肌肉血管内(图 2-10-b)。注射完后轻轻按摩注射部位,以助药物吸收。

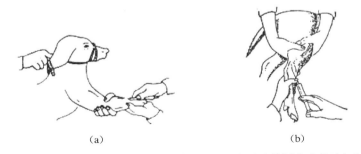

(a)　　　　　　　　　　　　　　(b)

图 2-10　前肢内侧皮下大静脉注射法(a)和犬后肢外侧小隐静脉(b)

第三节　实验动物标本采集方法

一、血液的采集

不同采血方法的选择,决定于实验的目的所需血量以及动物种类。凡用血量较少的实验如红、白细胞计数、血红蛋白的测定、血液涂片以及酶活性微量分析法等,可刺破组织取毛细血管的血。当需血量较多时可作静脉采血。静脉采血时,若需反复多次,应自远离心脏端静脉开始,以免发生栓塞而影响整条静脉。研究毒物对肺功能的影响、血液酸碱平衡、水盐代谢紊乱,需要比较静、动脉血氧分压、二氧化碳分压和血液 pH 值以及 K^+、Na^+、Cl^- 离子浓度,必须采取动脉血液。

(一) 大、小鼠采血法

1. 割(剪)尾采血

当所需血量很少时采用本法。固定动物并露出鼠尾。将尾部毛剪去后消毒,然后浸在 45℃左右的温水中数分钟,使尾部血管充盈。再将尾擦干,用锐器(刀或剪刀)割去尾尖 0.3～0.5 cm,让血液自由滴入盛器或用血红蛋白吸管吸取,采血结束,伤口消毒并压迫止血。也可在尾部作一横切口,割破尾动脉或静脉,收集血液的方法同上。每鼠一般可采血 10 余次左右。小鼠每次可取血 0.1 ml,大鼠 0.3～0.5 ml。采血占全血量的 10%不会对机体造成严重的不良影响。最大安全采血量:小鼠循环血量占体重的 6%,或 50～70 ml/kg,3～4 周后可以重新采集 1 次。如果需要很短时间反复采血,比如每天 1 次,每次的采血量不应超过全血的 1%。

2. 鼠尾刺血法

大鼠用血量不多时(仅做白细胞计数或血红蛋白检查),可采用本法。先将鼠尾用温水擦拭,再用酒精消毒和擦拭,使鼠尾充血。用 7 号或 8 号注射针头,刺入鼠尾静脉,拔出针头时即有血滴出,一次可采集 10～50 ml。如果长期反复取血,应先靠近鼠尾末端穿刺,以后再逐渐向近心端穿刺。

3. 眼眶静脉丛采血

采血者的左手拇、食两指从背部较紧地握住小鼠或大鼠的颈部(大鼠采血需带上纱手套),应防止动物窒息。当取血时左手拇指及食指轻轻压迫动物的颈部两侧,使眶后静脉丛充血。右手持接 7 号针头的 1 ml 注射器或长颈(3～4 cm)硬质玻璃滴管(毛细管内径 0.5～1.0 mm),使采血器与鼠面成 45°的夹角,由眼内角刺入,针头斜面先向眼球,刺入后再转 180°使斜面对着眼眶后界。刺入深度,小鼠约 2～3 mm,大鼠约 4～5 mm。当感到有阻力时即停止推进,同时,将针退出约 0.1～0.5 mm,边退边抽。若穿刺适当血液能自然流入毛细管中,当得到所需的血量后,即除去加在颈部的压力,同时,将采血器拔出,以防止术后穿刺孔出血。若技术熟练,用本法短期内可重复采血均无多大困难。左右两眼轮换更好。体重 20～25 g 的小鼠每次可采血 0.2～0.3 ml;体重 200～300 g 大鼠每次可采血 0.5～1.0 ml,可适用于某些生物化学项目的检验。

4. 断头取血

采血者的左手拇指和食指以背部较紧地握住大(小)鼠的颈部皮肤,并使动物头朝下倾的姿势。右手用剪刀猛剪鼠颈,约 1/2～4/5 的颈部前剪断,让血自由滴入盛器。小鼠可采血约 0.8～1.2 ml;大鼠约 5～10 ml。

5. 心脏采血

鼠类的心脏较小,且心率较快,心脏采血比较困难,故少用。若做开胸一次死亡采血,先将动物作深麻醉,打开胸腔,暴露心脏,用针头刺入右心室,吸取血液。小鼠可采血约 0.5～0.6 ml;大鼠约 0.8～1.2 ml。

6. 颈静脉采血

先将动物仰位固定,切开颈部皮肤,分离皮下结缔组织,使颈静脉充分暴露,可用注射器吸出血液。

7. 腹主动脉采血

最好先将动物麻醉,仰卧固定在手术架上,从腹正中线皮肤切开腹腔,使腹主动脉清楚暴露。用注射器吸出血液,防止溶血。或用无齿镊子剥离结缔组织,夹住动脉近心端,用尖头手术剪刀,剪断动脉,使血液喷入盛器。

8. 股动脉采血

先由助手握住动物,采血者左手拉直动物下肢,以搏动为指标,右手用注射器刺入血管。体重 15～20 g 小鼠采血约 0.2～0.8 ml,大鼠约 0.4～0.6 ml。

(二) 豚鼠采血法

1. 耳缘剪口采血

将耳消毒后,用锐器(刀或刀片)割破耳缘,在切口边缘涂抹 20% 枸橼酸钠溶液,阻止血凝,则血可自切口自动流出,进入盛器。操作时,使耳充血效果较好。此法能采血 0.5 ml 左右。

2. 心脏采血

取血前应探明心脏搏动最强部位,通常在胸骨左缘的正中,选心跳最显的部位作穿刺。针头宜稍细长些,以免发生手术后穿刺孔出血,其操作手法详见兔心脏采血。因豚鼠身体较小,一般由助手握住前后肢进行采血即可。成年豚鼠每周采血应不超过 10 ml 为宜。

3. 股动脉采血

将动脉仰位固定在手术台上,剪去腹股沟区的毛,麻醉后,局部用碘酒消毒。切开长约 2～3 cm 的皮肤,使股动脉暴露及分离。然后,用镊子提起股动脉,远端结扎,近端用止血钳夹住,在动脉中央剪一小孔,用无菌玻璃小导管或聚乙烯管插入,放开止血钳,血液即从导管口流出。一次可采血 10～20 ml。

4. 背中足静脉取血

助手固定动物,将其右或左膝关节伸直提到术者面前。术者将动物脚背面用酒精消毒,找出背中足静脉后,以左手的拇指和食指拉住豚鼠的趾端,右手将注射针刺入静脉。拔针后立即出血,呈半球状隆起。采血后,用纱布或脱脂棉压迫止血。反复采血时,两后肢可交替使用。

(三) 兔采血法

1. 耳静脉采血

本法为最常用的取血法之一,常作多次反复取血用。因此,保护耳缘静脉,防止发生栓塞特别重要。将兔放入仅露出头部及两耳的固定盒中,选耳静脉清晰的耳朵,将耳静脉部位的毛剪去,用 75% 酒精局部消毒,待干。用手指轻轻摩擦兔耳,使静脉扩张,用连有 5 号针头的注射器在耳缘静脉末端刺破血管待血液漏出取血或将针头逆血流方向刺入耳缘静脉取血,取血完毕用棉球压迫止血,此种采血法一次最多可采血 5～10 ml。

2. 耳中央动脉采血

将兔置于兔固定箱内,在兔耳的中央有一条较粗、颜色较鲜红的中央动脉,用左手固定兔耳,右手取注射器,在中央动脉的末端,沿着动脉平行地向心方向刺入动脉,即可见动脉血进入针筒,取血完毕后注意止血。但抽血时应注意,由于兔耳中央动脉容易发生痉挛性收缩,因此抽血前,必须先让兔耳充分充血,当动脉扩张,未发生痉挛性收缩之前立即进行抽血,如果等待时间过长,动脉经常会发生较长时间的痉挛性收缩。取血用的针头一般用 6 号针头,不要太细。针刺部位从中央动脉末端开始。不要在近耳根部取血,因耳根部软组织厚,血管位置略深,易刺透血管造成皮下出血,此法一次抽血可达 15 ml。

3. 心脏采血

将兔仰卧固定,在第三肋胸骨左缘 3 mm 处注射针垂直刺入心脏,血液随即进入针管。注意事项有:①动作宜迅速,以缩短在心脏内的留针时间和防止血液凝固;②如针头已进入心脏但抽不出血时,应将针头稍微后退一点;③在胸腔内针头不应左右摆动以防止伤及心、肺,一次可取血 20～25 ml。

4. 后肢胫部皮下静脉采血

将兔仰卧固定于兔固定板上,或由一人将兔固定好。剪去胫部被毛,在胫部上端股部扎以橡皮管,则在胫部外侧浅表皮下,可清楚见到皮下静脉。用左手两指固定好静脉,右手取带有 5(1/2)号针头的注射器内皮下静脉平行方向刺入血管,抽一下针栓,如血进入注射器,表示针头已刺入血管,即可取血。取完后必须用棉球压迫取血部位止血,时间要略长些,因此处不易止血。如止血不妥,可造成皮下血肿,影响连续多次取血,一次可取 2～5 ml。

5. 颈静脉、股静脉采血

先作股静脉和颈静脉暴露分离手术,注射器平行于血管,从股静脉下端向心方向刺入,徐徐抽动针栓即可取血。抽血完毕后要注意止血。股静脉较易止血,用纱布轻压取血部位即可。若连续多次取血,取血部位宜尽量选择靠离心端。颈静脉取血时,注射器由近心端(距颈静脉分支 2～3 cm 处)向头侧端顺血管平等方向刺入,使注射针一直引深至颈静脉分支叉处,即可取血。此处血管较粗,很容易取血,取血量也较多,取血完毕,拔出针头,用干纱布轻轻压迫取血部位也易止血。兔急性实验的静脉取血,用此法较方便,一次可取 10 ml 以上。

6. 颈动脉采血

固定好麻醉兔子,作颈动脉暴露分离手术及颈总动脉插管。取血时,放开夹在动脉近心端的动脉夹即可。

(四)狗采血法

1. 后肢外侧小隐静脉和前肢内侧皮下静脉采血

此法最常用,且方便。抽血前,将狗固定在狗架上或使狗侧卧,由助手将狗固定好。将抽血部位的毛剪去,碘酒消毒皮肤。采血者左手拇指和食指握紧剪毛区上部,使下肢静脉充盈,右手用连有 6 号或 7 号针头的注射器迅速穿刺入静脉,左手放松将针固定,以适当速度抽血(以无气泡为宜)。或将胶皮带绑在狗股部,或由助手握紧股部,即可,若仅需少量血液,可以不用注射器抽取,只需用针头直接刺入静脉,待血从针孔自然滴出,放入盛器或作涂片。

2. 股动脉采血

本法为采取狗动脉血最常用的方法。操作也较简便。稍加以训练的狗,在清醒状态下将狗卧位固定于狗解剖台上。伸展后肢向外伸直，暴露腹沟三角动脉搏动的部位，剪去被毛。用碘酒消毒。左手中指、食指探摸股动脉跳动部位，并固定好血管，右手取连有5(1/2)号针头的注射器，针头由动脉跳动处直接刺入血管，若刺入动脉一般可见鲜红血液流入注射器，有时还需微微转动一下针头或上下移动一下针头，方见鲜血流入。有时，会刺入静脉，必须重抽之。待抽血完毕，迅速拔出针头，用干药棉压迫止血2～3 min。

3. 心脏采血

本法最好在麻醉下进行，驯服的狗不麻醉也行。将固定在手术台上，前肢向背侧方向固定，暴露胸部，将左侧第3～5肋间的被毛剪去，用碘酒消毒皮肤。采血者用左手触摸左侧3～5肋间处，选择心跳最显处穿刺。一般选择胸骨左缘外1 cm第4肋间处。取连有6号针头的注射器，由上述部位进针，并向动物背侧方向垂直刺入心脏。采血者可随针接触心跳的感觉，随时调整刺入方向和深度，摆动的角度尽量小，避免损伤心肌过重，或造成胸腔大出血。当针头正确刺入心脏时，血即可进入注射器，可抽取多量血液。

4. 耳缘静脉采血

本法宜取少量血液作血常规或微量酶活力检查等。稍有训练的狗不必绑嘴，剪去耳尖部被毛，即可见耳缘静脉，手法基本与兔采血相同。

5. 颈静脉采血

狗不需麻醉，经训练的狗不需固定，未经训练的狗应予固定。取侧卧位，剪去颈部被毛约10 cm×3 cm范围，用碘酒、酒精消毒皮肤。将狗颈部拉直，头尽量后抑。用左手拇指压住颈静脉入胸部位的皮肤。使颈静脉怒张，右手取连有6号针头的注射器。针头沿血管平行方向向心端刺往前血管。由于此静脉在皮下易滑动，针刺时除用左手固定好血管外，刺入要准确。取血后注意压迫止血。采用此法一次可采较多量的血。

二、尿液的采集

实验动物的尿液常用代谢笼采集，也可通过其他装置来采集。

（一）代谢笼采集尿液

代谢笼用于收集实验动物自然排出的尿液，是一种特别设计的为采集实验动物各种排泄物的密封式饲养笼，有的代谢笼除可收集尿液外，又可收集粪便和动物呼出的CO_2。一般简单的代谢笼主要用来收集尿液。

（二）导尿法采集尿液

施行导尿术，较适宜于犬、猴等大型动物。一般不需要麻醉，导尿时将实验动物仰卧固定，用甘油润滑导尿管。对雄性动物，操作员用一只手握住阴茎，另一只手将阴茎包皮向下，暴露龟头，使尿道口张开，将导尿管缓慢插入，导尿管推进到尿道膜部时有抵抗感，此时注意动作轻柔，继续向膀胱推进导尿管，即有尿液流出。雌性动物尿道外口在阴道前庭，导尿时于阴道前庭腹侧将导尿管插入阴道外口，其后操作同雄性动物导尿术。

用导尿法导尿可采集到没有污染的尿液。如果严格执行无菌操作，可收集到无菌尿液。

（三）输尿管插管采集尿液

一般用于要求精确计量单位时间内实验动物排尿量的实验。剖腹后，将膀胱牵拉至腹腔外，暴露膀胱底两侧的输尿管。在两侧输尿管近膀胱处用线分别结扎，于输尿管结扎处上方剪一小口，向肾脏方向分别插入充满生理盐水的插管，用线结扎固定插管，即可见尿液从插管滴出,可以收集。

(四)压迫膀胱采集尿液

实验人员用手在实验动物下腹部加压,手法既轻柔又有力。当增加的压力使实验动物膀胱括约肌松弛时,尿液会自动流出,即行收集。

(五)穿刺膀胱采集尿液

实验动物麻醉固定后,剪去下腹部耻骨联合之上,腹正中线两侧的被毛,消毒后用注射针头接注射器穿刺。取钝角进针,针头穿过皮肤后稍微改变角度,以避免穿刺后漏尿,然后刺向膀胱方向,边缓慢进针边回抽,直到抽到尿液为止。

(六)剖腹采集尿液

按上述穿刺膀胱采集尿液法做术前准备,其皮肤准备范围应更大。剖腹暴露膀胱,直视下穿刺膀胱抽取尿液。也可于穿刺前用无齿镊夹住部分膀胱壁,从镊子下方的膀胱壁进针抽尿。

(七)提鼠采集尿液(即反射排尿法)

鼠类被人抓住尾巴提起即出现排尿反射,以小鼠的这种反射最明显。可以利用这一反射收集尿液。当鼠类被提起尾巴排尿后,尿滴挂在尿道外口附近的被毛上,不会马上流走,操作人员应迅速用吸管或玻璃管接住尿滴。

(八)膀胱插管法采集尿液

腹部手术同输尿管插管。将膀胱翻出腹外后,用丝线结扎膀胱颈部,阻断它同尿道的通路。然后在膀胱顶部避开血管剪一小口,插入膀胱漏斗,用丝线做以荷包缝合固定。漏斗最好正对着输尿管的入口处。注意不要紧贴膀胱后壁而堵塞输尿管。下端接橡皮管插入带刻度的容器内以采集尿液。

三、分泌液的采集

(一)阴道分泌物的采集

适于观察阴道角质化上皮细胞。

1. 滴管冲洗法

用消毒滴管吸取少量生理盐水仔细、反复冲洗被检雌性动物阴道,将冲洗液吸出滴在载玻片上晾干后染色镜检。也可直接将冲洗液置于低倍显微镜下观察,根据细胞类型变化鉴别实验动物动情周期中的不同时期。

2. 棉拭子法

用消毒棉拭子旋转插入动物阴道内,然后在阴道内轻轻转动几下后取出,即可进行涂片镜检。有的动物如大、小鼠等,阴道液较少,取其阴道液时,可用先浸湿后又挤尽无菌生理盐水的棉拭子取阴道液,这种棉拭子比干棉拭子容易插入阴道。对体型较大的实验动物,也可先按摩或刺激其阴部,而后再采集其阴道液。

3. 刮取法

用光滑的玻璃小勺或牛角制的小刮片慢慢插入阴道内,在阴道壁轻轻刮取一点阴道内含物,进行涂片镜检。

(二)精液的采集

1. 人工阴道套采精液法

本法适用于犬、猪、羊等大动物,采用特制的人工阴道套套在实验动物阴茎上采集精液。

采精时,一手捏住阴道套,套住雄性动物的阴茎,以完全套住雄性动物的阴茎为佳,插入阴道套后,若实验动物发出低叫声,表明已经射精。此时可取下阴道套,拆下采精瓶,取出精液,迅速做有关检查。

2. 阴道栓采精法

本法是将阴道栓涂片染色,镜检凝固的精液。阴道栓是雄性大、小鼠的精液和雌性阴道分泌物混合,在雌鼠阴道内凝结而成白色稍透明、圆锥形的栓状物,一般交配后2～4 h即可在雌鼠阴道口形成,并可在阴道停留12～24 h。

3. 其他采精液法

将发情的雌性动物放在雄性动物一起,当雄性动物被刺激发情后,立即将雄性动物分开,再用人工法刺激其射精。也可按摩雄性动物的生殖器或用电流等物理方法刺激雄性动物的阴茎或其他性敏感区,使雄性动物被刺激发情,直至射精,用采精瓶采集射出的精液。

(三)乳汁的采集

用按摩挤奶收集乳汁的方法适合犬、猪、羊等大型动物乳汁的采集。选用哺乳期的实验动物,在早上采集乳汁量最多,用手指轻轻按摩实验动物乳头,使乳汁自然流出,如乳汁不能自然流出,可张开手掌从乳房基底部朝乳头方向按摩、挤压整个乳房,即可挤出乳汁。

四、消化液的采集

(一)唾液

1. 直接抽取法

在急性实验中,可用吸管直接插入动物口腔或唾液腺导管抽吸唾液,此法非常简单,但从口腔抽吸唾液会有杂质混入。

2. 制造腮腺瘘法

在慢性实验中,收集狗的唾液,要用外科手术方法将腮腺导管开口移向体外,即以腮腺导管为中心,切成一直径约2～3 cm的圆形黏膜片,将此黏膜片,与周围组织分开,穿过皮肤切口引到颊外,将带有导管开口的黏膜片与周围的皮肤缝合,腮腺分泌的唾液就流出颊外。这种方法可以收集到较纯净的唾液。

(二)胃液

1. 直接收集胃液法

急性实验时,先将动物麻醉,将灌胃管经口插入胃内,在灌胃管的出口连一注射器,用此注射器可收集到胃液,此法适用于狗等大型动物。如是大鼠,需手术剖腹,从幽门端向胃内插入一塑料管,再由口腔经食道将一塑料管插入前胃,用pH7.5、35℃左右的生理盐水,以12 ml/h的流速灌胃,收集流出液,进行分析。

2. 制备胃瘘法

在慢性实验中,收集胃液多用胃瘘法,如全胃瘘法、巴氏小胃瘘法、海氏小胃瘘法等。制备小胃是将动物的胃分离出一小部分,缝合起来形成小胃,主胃与小胃互不相通,主胃进行正常消化,从小胃可收集到纯净的胃液。应用该法,可以在动物清醒状态下反复采集胃液。

(三)胰液和胆汁

在动物实验中,主要是通过对胰总管和胆总管的插管而获得胰液或胆汁。狗的胰总管开口于十二指肠降部,在紧靠肠壁处切开胰管,结扎固定并与导管相连,即可见无色的胰液流入导管。大鼠的胰管与胆管汇集于一个总管,在其入肠处插管固定,并在近肝门处结扎和另行插管,可分别收集到胰液和胆汁。有时也可通过制备胰瘘和胆囊瘘来获得胰液和胆汁。

四、实验动物的安死术

实验动物的处死必须遵循实验动物的伦理要求和动物福利法按照人道主义原则处死实验动物。

1."安死术"的概念:即安乐死术,是指以人道的方法处死动物过程。在处死动物的过程中尽量减少动物的惊慌、焦虑,使其安静地、无痛苦地死亡。

2.安死术的常用方法

(1)颈椎脱位法

是将实验动物的颈椎脱臼,断离脊髓 致死,为大、小鼠最常用的处死方法。

(2)空气栓塞法

处死兔、猫、犬常用此法,兔、猫为 20～40 ml,犬为 80～150 ml。

(3)过量麻醉处死

此法多用于处死大鼠、豚鼠和家兔,吸入乙醚或腹腔注射巴比妥钠。

(4)二氧化碳吸入法

让实验动物吸入大量 CO_2 等气体而中毒死亡。

3.采用安死术必须符合的标准

① 死时无惊恐、疼痛表现;

② 使其在最短时间内失去意识,迅速死亡;

③ 方法可靠且可重复;

④ 对操作人员安全;

⑤ 采用的方法要与研究要求和目的一致;

⑥ 对观察者和操作者的情绪影响最小;

⑦ 对环境的影响最小;

⑧ 需要的机械设备简单、价廉、易操作;

⑨ 处死动物地点应远离并与动物房隔开。

第四节　常用手术器械

一、哺乳动物实验需用手术器械

常用的有剪刀、止血钳、皮钳、镊子等,根据不同的实验要求选择合适的手术器械(图2-11)。

1.剪刀

常用的有直剪刀、弯剪刀和眼科剪刀 3 种。弯剪刀用来剪被毛;直剪刀剪开皮肤,皮下组织,腹白线等,禁用手术剪剪骨骼等坚硬组织;眼科剪

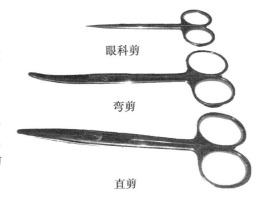

眼科剪

弯剪

直剪

用于剪破血管,剪断神经,要注意保护眼科剪的尖端,不能随意剪坚韧的组织、皮肤、线团等。

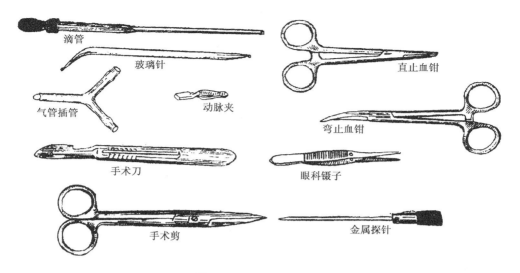

滴管
玻璃针
直止血钳
气管插管
动脉夹
弯止血钳
手术刀
眼科镊子
手术剪
金属探针

图 2-11　常用手术器械

持剪方法是以拇指和环指分别插入剪柄的左右两环,中指放在环指的前外方剪柄上,食指轻压在剪柄和刀口交界的轴节处。

2．止血钳

止血钳有长、短、弯、直等多种规格。主要用于止血和钝性分离组织,用于止血时尖端应与组织垂直,夹住出血血管断端,尽量少夹附近组织。小号止血钳又叫"蚊式钳",适用于分离小血管及神经周围的结缔组织。止血钳头端齿槽床咬合面有细齿,便于钳夹固定皮肤组织等,两柄之间有扣齿,扣上之后止血钳头端不易松开。

持钳方法与持剪方法相同,放开时用拇指和无名指轻轻上下交错即可。

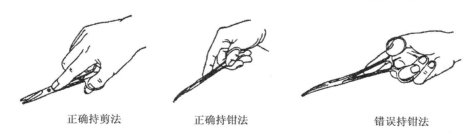

正确持剪法
正确持钳法
错误持钳法

图 2-12　持钳(剪)的方法

3．皮钳

皮钳和止血钳的区别在于齿槽床,皮钳的齿槽床扁而宽,对组织的压榨较血管钳轻,所以用来钳夹或牵拉皮肤,也可夹在切口的边缘用于打开手术野。

4．镊子

镊子分为有齿镊和无齿镊两种,也有长、短、弯、直之分。有齿镊用于夹持较坚韧的组织,如皮肤、筋膜、肌腱等,无齿镊用于夹持细软组织,如皮下组织、脂肪、黏膜等。眼科镊可在动静脉插管时扩张切口便于导管插入。

持镊方法是用拇指、食指和中指把持镊子的中部。

5. 动脉夹

动脉夹有大、小之分。小动脉夹主要用于夹闭血管,暂时阻断血流,便于进行血管插管。大动脉夹用于固定头皮静脉针,也可以用来代替手指阻断兔耳缘静脉血流,使血管充盈以便进行耳缘静脉穿刺。

6. 气管插管

气管插管为"Y"形管。急性动物实验时做气管切开插入气管插管,以保证呼吸道通畅。有时根据实验需要,在气管插管的"Y"形分叉的两端接上 2～3 cm 的橡胶管。

7. 膀胱插管

膀胱插管分为体内端和体外端,两端之间连接橡胶软管。体内端为直玻璃管,插入到膀胱内的部分略微膨出称为壶腹部,紧接着上方有一相对狭窄段称为颈部。壶腹部插入到膀胱后在玻璃管颈部打结固定。

8. 其他

小勾子、滴管、玻璃针、针头等根据实验需要选用。

二、蛙类实验需用手术器械

1. 剪刀

大号手术剪用来剪骨骼、肌肉、皮肤、内脏。眼科剪用于剪神经和血管等细软组织。

2. 金属探针

用于破坏蛙或蟾蜍的脑和脊髓。

3. 镊子

有齿镊用来夹住蛙的脊柱,无齿镊用于夹伤坐骨神经。

4. 玻璃分针

用于分离血管和神经等组织。

5. 蛙钉

为固定蛙腿的专用品,没有时也可用大头针固定。

6. 蛙板

用于固定蛙类动物,周围是木板,中间为玻璃板。可用蛙钉或大头针将蛙腿固定于木板上,以利用操作,将肌肉和暴露的神经尽量置于用任氏液湿润的玻璃面,可减低损伤,保持兴奋性。

第五节　常　用　仪　器

一、RM6240 EC 多道生理信号采集处理系统

1. 仪器简介

RM6240 EC 多道生理信号采集处理系统是成都仪器厂研制的新一代医学实验设备。该系统是综合应用最新多媒体计算机技术,先进的电子技术和数字信号处理技术,基于现代医学机能实验的要求,总结长期医学实验教学的经验研制而成的最新产品。

系统由硬件和软件两部分组成。硬件包括外置程控放大器、数据采集板、数据线及各种信号输入输出线。其面板上设置有外接信号输入插座、刺激器输出插座、记滴及监听插座（图2-13）。

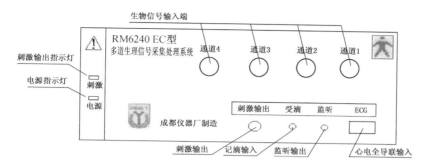

图 2-13　RM6240 EC 多道生理信号采集仪面板示意图

（1）通道输入接口

通道是模拟信号输入、处理放大、转换成数字信号并被显示记录的物理通路。一般多通道生理信号采集处理系统有4个物理通道，可同时处理放大和记录4路信号。RM6240 EC 4个物理通道输入接口采用5芯航空插座，插头与插座有对应的凹凸槽。

（2）刺激输出接口

输出刺激电压或电流，刺激波形为方波。

（3）受滴器输入接口

用于插入受滴器，记录液体的滴数。该接口也可用于外触发。

（4）监听输出接口

接有源音箱可监听第1通道信号的声音。

（5）ECG 接口

接 IEC 标准导连线，可观察记录12导联心电图。

软件主要由 RM6240. exe 及多个实验子模块组成。系统使用 Windows 风格的中文图形界面，操作简便易学。软件与硬件协调工作，实现系统的多种功能。主要操作界面如图2-14所示。

（6）菜单条

显示顶层菜单项。选择其中的一项即可弹出其子菜单。

（7）工具条

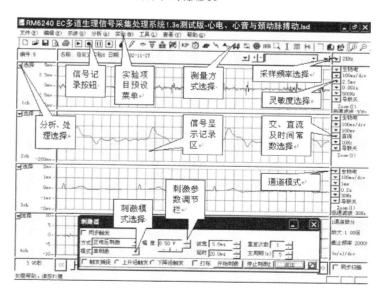

图 2-14　RM6240 EC 多道生理信号采集系统软件窗

工具条的位置处于菜单条的下方。工具条提供了仪器基本功能的快捷按钮。菜单条中最常用的指令,都能在工具条中找到对应的图标(只需鼠标直接点击即可)。在操作工具条时,一旦鼠标指向某图标即会弹出其指令名称。

(8) 参数设置区

位于窗口的右侧。有"采样频率"及各通道的"通道模式""灵敏度""时间常数""滤波""扫描速度"等参数,用鼠标选择各功能键可调节各通道的实验参数。本系统每个通道都是多功能放大器,均可作血压放大器和生物电放大器。

(9) 数据显示区

实验数据以波形的形式显示于该区域内。

(10) 标尺及处理区

该区显示各通道的通道号及对应信号量纲的标尺。鼠标点击"处理"按钮,弹出菜单,有对应通道定标、标记显示、分析测量、数据处理等功能选项。

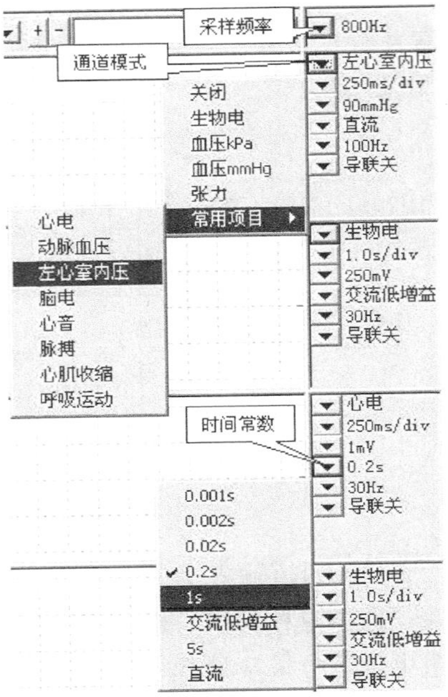

图 2-15 通道模式和时间常数设置

(11) 刺激器

程控刺激器为一弹出式浮动窗口,该刺激器可满足各种实验刺激的需要。

2. 主要参数

任何实验,只要生物信号无问题,要取得好的实验效果,关键是实验参数(用系统界面右边控制参数区的按键调节)的设置,实际上取决于选择合适的"采集频率""通道模式""扫描速度""灵敏度""时间常数""滤波频率"。当有 50 Hz 交流干扰时,还应将示波菜单中的"50 Hz 陷波开"打开(当所采集的信号频率本身处于 50 Hz 附近时不宜打开"50 Hz 陷波")。这里重点将上述几个实验参数逐一介绍(图 2-15)。

(1) 通道模式

用来选择放大器的工作模式,本系统的放大器是全功能程控放大器,通过通道模式选择各通道的放大器均可成为生物电放大器、血压放大器、桥式放大器、温度放大器、呼吸流量放大器等,如作血压实验时,应选择血压模式,并根据习惯选择血压单位。根据已知输入信号的特性,系统可通过软件工具栏中的创建新量纲功能添加或删除放大器的工作模式。本系统预先设置了生物电、血压(对应 YP100 型压力换能器)、体温(对应 CW100 型温度换能器)、温度(对应 CPT100 型温度换能器)、呼吸流量(对应 HX200 型呼吸流量换能器)等通道模式,并已打开了生物电和血压模式。在通道模式中有常用项目选择,用于在实验中迅速设定常用实验的参数,此后只需对采集频率及灵敏度根据需要稍作调整即可。但对于不同的实验对象,不同的信号频率应适当调整滤波参数。通道模式中的交流低增益模式是时间常数为 1s 的低放大倍数交流模式,用于某些特殊场合,若需时间常数更小的交流低增益模式,可在此模式下再结合数字滤波的高通滤波来实现。

(2) 采集频率

系统采集数据的频率,如采集频率 100 kHz 表示系统以 100 000 点/秒的速度采集数据。由于计算机画一个波形是以若干点组成的,所以采集频率应高于信号频率若干倍才能分辨出有效信号。信号频率越高,需要的采集频率就越高。但在实际应用中,采集频率也不是越高越好,对于低频的信号,选择过高的采集频率非但对显示的波形没有改善,反而会占用过大的存储空间。本系统共有 21 档采集频率(从 1 Hz～100 kHz),在每一档采集频率均有若干档扫描速度供选择(在同一档采集频率下,扫描速度可有 1 000 倍的调节量),亦即在同一采集频率下,各通道的扫描速度独立可调,通道间的扫描速度可达 1 000 倍的差别。如选择了同步扫描(在界面右下角),则各通道扫描速度均相同,只能同步调节。在同样的扫描速度下,只要信号波形好,选择低的采样频率有助于减小记录的文件空间。但对于频谱丰富的信号,选择的采集频率过低,则会丢失信号的高频成分。如做神经放电实验时,尽管选择的扫描速度并不高,但仍需要选择足够高的采集频率。故采集频率的物理意义可比喻为采集卡的频率响应。

（3）扫描速度

计算机显示波形的扫描速度,如 1 s/div 表示水平方向一个大格代表 1 s 时间,相当于描笔式记录仪的走纸速度。和描笔式记录仪不同的是,本系统的扫描速度不是唯一的。例如:当采集频率为 200 Hz 时,可选择 100 ms/div 的扫描速度,但在采集频率为 8 kHz 时,也可选择 100 ms/div 的扫描速度。但二者的物理意义是不同的,前者的频率响应低,后者的频率响应高,用前者无法观察神经放电现象,用后者则可观察。而对观察脉搏波这种低频信号来说,二者效果差不多,但前者的数据量仅为后者的 1/40,显然用前者更有助于节约数据存储空间。

（4）灵敏度

物理意义与描笔式记录仪的灵敏度相同,用于选择放大器的放大倍数。当观察到的信号太大或太小时,应相应地减小或提高灵敏度(图 2-16)。

（5）时间常数

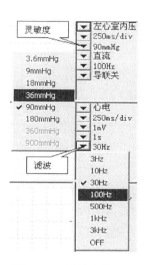

图 2-16　灵敏度和滤波设置

物理意义与描笔式记录仪的时间常数相同。时间常数用于调节放大器高通滤波器的时间常数,它与高通滤波器的低频截止频率成反比关系。高通滤波器用来滤除信号的低频成份,信号的有效成分频率越高,应选择的时间常数越小,如作神经实验时,因有效信号频率高,应该选择小的时间常数,将低频成分隔离掉,以有助于基线的稳定。有效信号频率低时,应选择高的时间常数或选择直流,如作胃肠电实验时选择 5 s 的时间常数,作张力实验时选择直流等等。时间常数代表放大器低频滤波的程度,如 1、0.1、0.01、0.001 s 分别对应放大器的下限截止频率为 0.16、1.6、16、160 Hz。时间常数越小,下限截止频率就越高,亦即对低频成分的滤波程度越大。当选择直流时,放大器不作高通滤波,此时放大器将信号中的交流和直流成分均作了放大。

（6）滤波频率

物理意义与描笔式记录仪的滤波频率相同,用来滤除信号的高频成分。当信号有效成分频率较低时,应选择低的滤波频率,以滤除高频干扰。如观察脉搏波时,选择 10 Hz 的滤波,代表此时放大器的上限截止频率为 10 Hz,可将 10 Hz 以上的各种干扰滤掉。

3. 操作流程

在本实验课程中,使用本系统的基本操作流程图 2-17:

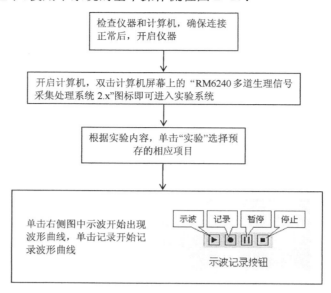

图 2-17 基本操作流程图

（1）打标记

在实验过程中,对实验对象的反应及各种处理进行标注,有利于准确的进行实验数据的整理。快捷的对数据进行浏览和标记搜索,可以大大提高实验数据整理的效率。字符的标记可以在图 2-18 所示的功能区实现(图 2-18)。

一般实验项目中用到的标记均已经在系统中预存,使用时只需要在记录状态点击"打标记"即可在每个通道波形上同时记录下所加标记名称。如果没有找到所需字符,可以自行添加。

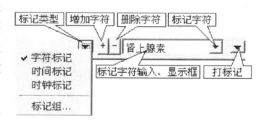

图 2-18 字符标记功能区

此外,在记录、暂停或分析状态用鼠标右键在各个通道波形的任意位置加入标记。当右键周围已有标记时,系统会弹出一个移动菜单,可以进行修改、删除和打标操作。

（2）数据编辑

在"编辑"菜单选择"数据编辑"或在工具栏点击"数据编辑"工具"I",系统即进入数据编辑状态,并在屏幕右上角弹出浮动的数据编辑工具小窗口(图 2-19)。

此选项便于在通道中直接对波形(数据)进行剪切。选取此项指令后,按住鼠标左键并拖动鼠标即可选取任意范围需要编辑的波形(选中的波形背景颜色为黑色),此时,可通过以下命令对波形进行处理,以便保存和打印。注意:数据编辑改变了所采集的原始数据位置,如仅需剪贴和编辑图形,可用鼠标捕捉功能将图形复制到"Word"或波形图板中编辑。

退出该命令时可再次点击工具"I"或用"Esc"键。

"选取数据段"操作步骤:

① 将鼠标移到欲选取的波形起始处,按下鼠标左键;

② 按住鼠标左键并左右拖动鼠标至欲编辑波形的末端(鼠标过处的波形被涂黑);

③ 释放鼠标左键,则已涂黑的波形段数据被视为已选取的数据段。

当无效数据段较少时,用以下两个命令可很方便的保留有效数据。

剪切:用此命令可将当前被选取的数据段删除。

撤销:用于恢复上一步数据剪切工作。注意:该功能只能撤销一个步骤。

当有效数据段较少时,用以下两个命令可很方便的保留有效数据。

选择剪接区域:选取一段数据后点击该键,以确定一段数据。反复操作即可选取多段欲保留的数据段。

显示剪接结果:当选取完欲保留数据段后点击该键,即可将所选取的所有数据段自动连接并显示。

当需要取消所有的编辑,数据恢复到原始状态时,用"还原"键。该功能主要是为了避免误操作时将有效数据段除掉。

当需要观测剪切或剪接数据时产生的接点位置时,用"显示连接点标记"。

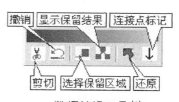

图 2-19　数据编辑工具窗口

二、752N 型分光光度计

分光光度计分析法是基于不同分子结构的物质对光的选择性吸收而建立的分析方法。

分光光度计的基本原理是溶液中的物质在光的照射激发下,产生了对光的吸收效应,物质对光的吸收是具有选择性的。各种不同的物质都具有其各自的吸收光谱,因此当某单色光通过溶液时,其能量就会被吸收而减弱,光能量减弱的程度和物质的浓度有一定的比例关系,也即符合于比色原理——比耳定律。

$$\tau = I/I_0$$
$$\log I_0 /I = KCL$$
$$A = KCL$$

其中:τ 为透射比;I_0 为入射光强度;I 为透射光强度;A 为吸光度;K 为吸收系数;L 为溶液的光径长度;C 为溶液的浓。

从以上公式可以看出,当入射光、吸收系数和溶液的光径长度不变时,透射光是根据溶液的浓度而变化的。实验中所用 752 N 紫外可见分光光度计的基本原理是根据上述之物理光学现象而设计的。

紫外可见分光光度计波长范围 200～800 nm,能在紫外、可见光谱区域对样品物质作定性和定量的分析。该仪器可广泛地应用于医药卫生、临床检验、生物化学、石油化工、环境保护、质量控制等部门,是理化实验室常用的分析仪器之一。仪器使用可按以下步骤进行。

① 调波长预热:插上电源插头,把波长旋钮旋至所测样品要求的波长,打开电源开关,

预热 30 min。

② 调零：将装有对照溶液和样品溶液的比色皿依次放入比色架；光路对准对照溶液比色皿。将仪器面板上"A/T/C/F"键设置为透射比"T%"挡，打开光门，按"▽/0%"键，使数值为"000.0"

③ 调 100%：关上光门，按"△/0A 100%"键，使数值显示为"100.0"。重复（2）、（3）步骤。

④ 测量：将仪器键盘上"A/T/C/F"键设置为"Abs."挡，此时显示 000.0，即对照溶液的吸光度为 0。依次移动比色皿，使样品溶液置于光路中，显示的数值即为对应样品溶液的吸光度。

⑤ 清洗：清洗比色皿。放好干燥剂。

⑥ 关机：使用完毕，关闭电源开关，罩上防尘罩。

三、FP 640 火焰光度计

利用火焰提供的热能使钾钠原子吸收能量后跃迁至上一个能量级，当它回落到正常能量级时，就要释放能量，这个释放的能量具有光谱特征，即在一定的波长范围。钾钠激发的特征光谱不同，配上不同的滤光片，就可以进行定性测试。焰色的强度又正比于溶液中所含原子的溶度，用仪器检测其光谱能量的强弱，进而判断物质中该元素含量的高低。这类仪器称之为火焰光度计。

火焰光度计本身无法得出被测元素的绝对浓度值。因此，必须首先制备标准溶液，进行检测标定，绘制标准曲线，然后对未知溶液进行测定。

1. 使用步骤

（1）开机测试

① 检查雾化

ⓐ 按下电源开关，启动空气压缩机，压力表上升至 0.15 MPa 左右。

ⓑ 打开进样开关，将吸管插入蒸馏水中，蒸馏水随吸管进入雾化室，不久废液皿内流出溶液，雾化正常。如果排水不畅，水积聚在雾化室里内，用手指反复挤压雾化室的乳胶管，直到排水畅通。

② 点火预热

ⓐ 打开液化气钢瓶上的开关（逆时针）；

ⓑ 向下按住燃气阀旋钮，从关闭位置左转 90°，按住不放就能点着火，点着后手指向里推一下再放手；

ⓒ 点火完成，再把燃气阀向左转（此时不要往里推）一直到不能转为止；

ⓓ 调节微调阀控制火苗大小；

ⓔ 预热 30 min 后测试。

③ 定标

ⓐ 显示一位小数，用面板显示屏下方薄膜按键调节；

ⓑ 进样吸管插入重蒸馏水，旋转面板"L"旋钮，使 K、Na 显示"0.0"；

ⓒ 进样吸管插入标准溶液 8 μg/ml，旋转面板"L"旋钮，使 K、Na 显示"8.0"；

ⓓ 进样吸管插入标准溶液 20 μg/ml，旋转面板"H"旋钮，使 K、Na 显示"20.0"；

ⓔ 重复 c、d 步骤。

④ 测试

进样吸管插入样品中,显示稳定后读数记录。

（2）关机步骤

① 关机前,在燃烧状态下进蒸馏水 5 min 清洗;

② 先关液化气钢瓶开关;

③ 再关燃气阀,微调阀不要关,下次开机点火仪器能保持原有的火苗大小;

④ 切断仪器和空气压缩机的电源。

2．注意事项

（1）仪器与液化气钢瓶周围不能摆放易燃易爆物品。实验环境必须通风良好。

（2）操作过程中,燃烧室与烟囱罩都是非常烫,不能将身体靠近或用手接触。

（3）每次测试完,应有 5 min 左右时间蒸馏水清洗。即进样吸管放在蒸馏水中同正常工作一样燃烧 5 min,循环清洗雾化室和燃烧头。

（4）平时进样吸管放在蒸馏水中。

（5）样品中不能含有颗粒状物质、动物毛发等。

（林琳　贺广远　陈晨　刘桦）

第三章 实验部分

实验一 实验动物手术基本操作技术

【实验目的】

（1）介绍机能实验学的特点和重要性；

（2）熟悉机能实验室各项规章制度和要求；

（3）掌握机能实验学的基本操作和要求；

（4）学习实验报告的正确撰写。

【实验材料】

（1）器材：金属器材；非金属器材。见表 3-1。

表 3-1　实验器材

金属器材（金属盘）		非金属器材（塑料盘）	
品名	数量	品名	数量
组织剪（直、弯）	2	头皮针	1
巾钳	4	玻璃分针	2
止血钳	3	粗棉绳	4
动脉夹	2	细棉绳	1
眼科剪	1	丝线	3
眼科镊	1	棉线	1
注射器针头	1	羽毛	1
非金属器材（塑料盘）		气管插管	1
品名	数量	动脉插管	1
搪瓷缸	1	膀胱插管	1
纱布	4	塑料杯	1
		注射器（20 ml；2 ml）	2

（2）药品：25%乌拉坦；1%肝素。

【实验对象】

家兔。

【实验步骤】

(一) 术前准备

(1) 抓兔:一只手抓住家兔颈背部皮肤,另一只手托其臀部。

(2) 称重:将家兔置于台秤进行称重。如家兔移动,可以通过轻轻抚摸其背部使之安静,以便称重。

(3) 麻醉:将家兔置于兔箱或手术台上,仔细辨认家兔的耳缘静脉,并除去覆于皮肤表面的兔毛,将 25%乌拉坦(4 ml/kg,1 g/kg)缓慢注射入耳缘静脉,通过下述 4 种指标判断麻醉深度。

疼痛反射:用止血钳夹住家兔脚趾会产生疼痛反应,引起肢体回缩,表示麻醉深度不足;如果肢体不回缩,表明家兔疼痛反射消失。

角膜反射:清醒状态的动物在用柔软的羽毛轻触角膜时会引起眨眼动作(角膜反射)。如果角膜反射消失,表明麻醉深度已经适宜进行手术。

肌肉张力:牵拉家兔四肢以检查肌肉张力。若肌肉张力高表明麻醉深度不足。如果四肢明显处于放松状态,则表明麻醉深度已达到手术要求。

心肺功能及体温监测:动物进入麻醉状态后,将出现呼吸频率减慢,心输出量减少,从而导致血液运输氧气减少,血压下降,组织血供减少,体温下降。

(4) 固定:仰卧位固定家兔于手术台上。

(二) 手术步骤

1. 颈部手术

(1) 剪毛:用弯组织剪剪去颈前部兔毛。

(2) 皮肤切口:用直组织剪于颈部正中做一 5～7 cm 长的切口,再用 4 把手术巾钳沿着对角线方向,向两侧将皮肤拉开。

(3) 分离皮下组织:在皮下组织做一类似皮肤上的切口,将皮下组织与肌肉层分离。

(4) 分离颈前肌肉:用两把止血钳交替分离颈前部肌肉,钝性分离、暴露气管。

(5) 气管插管:用弯止血钳分离气管与食管,在甲状软骨下 2～3 cm 处切开气管(倒 T 形切口),往肺脏方向插入气管插管并固定。

(6) 分离右侧颈动脉鞘内容物:仔细区分颈动脉鞘内的 3 根神经:迷走神经最粗;减压神经最细;颈交感神经居中。用玻璃分针将它们分离,并用不同颜色的丝线进行标记;最后分离该侧颈总动脉并用棉线标记。血管和神经的分离应操作轻柔,而且应首先分离最细的减压神经。不可用金属器械分离神经。

(7) 左侧颈总动脉插管:将左侧颈总动脉游离 2 cm,其远心端处用棉线结扎,近心端用动脉夹夹闭。用眼科剪在近颈总动脉远心端处剪一切口,向心脏方向插入颈总动

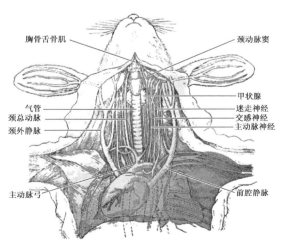

图 3-1　兔颈部和胸部解剖

脉插管,固定动脉插管。做颈总动脉插管术前,首先需实施抗凝血处理:全身肝素化——家兔耳缘静脉注射1%肝素;局部肝素化——家兔动脉插管中必须充盈有肝素液。在将颈总动脉插管与压力换能器连接之前,切勿松开动脉夹。

2. 上腹部手术

上腹正中剪开皮肤和分离皮下组织,认真寻找辨别腹白线后沿腹白线剪开腹壁肌肉层,并打开腹膜,暴露剑突。用蚊式钳(小号弯止血钳)小心分离胸骨与膈小肌;剪断胸骨,游离膈小肌后用一系着棉线的小钩钩住剑突(图3-2)。

3. 下腹部手术

耻骨联合上方正中剪开皮肤和皮下组织,沿腹白线剪开腹壁肌肉层,打开腹腔,暴露膀胱。

在膀胱顶部剪一个0.5 cm长的切口,插入膀胱插管,用棉线结扎固定膀胱插管。

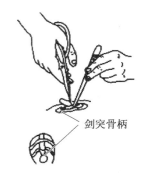

剑突骨柄

图 3-2　游离剑突的方法

【注意事项】

(1)乌拉坦耳缘静脉注射时要慢,否则家兔会因呼吸抑制而死亡。
(2)血管和神经的分离应操作轻柔,避免用金属器械分离神经。

【问题讨论】

(1)通过本次手术操作的学习,应如何进行输尿管插管以记录家兔尿量?
(2)外科手术为什么要规范化操作?

（戴小牛）

实验二　不同给药剂量对药物作用的影响

【实验目的】

(1)掌握小鼠的正确捉拿及腹腔注射给药方法;
(2)观察不同剂量的异戊巴比妥钠对小鼠作用的差异。

【实验原理】

异戊巴比妥钠对中枢神经系统有普遍性的抑制作用,随剂量增加可以相继出现动物的镇静、催眠、抗惊厥和麻醉作用。中等剂量的异戊巴比妥钠可引起小鼠催眠效应,睡眠以小鼠翻正反射消失为确定指标。翻正反射是指正常动物可以保持站立姿势,如将动物推倒或翻转,它可以迅速翻正,恢复站立,此种反射称为翻正反射。

【实验材料】

(1)器材:钟罩,天平,注射器(1 ml)。
(2)药品:0.3%和0.9%异戊巴比妥钠溶液。

【实验对象】

昆明系小鼠 2 只,体重 18～22 g/只。

【实验步骤】

(1) 取小鼠 2 只,称重并观察正常活动。分别腹腔注射 0.3% 的异戊巴比妥钠溶液(30 mg/kg)和 0.9% 的异戊巴比妥钠溶液(90 mg/kg),记录给药时间并观察小鼠活动情况。

(2) 观察项目:翻正反射消失。判断标准:用药后小鼠如果能维持四肢朝上时间 ≥ 1 min,就判断为翻正反射消失阳性。

(3) 实验结果填入表 3-2。

表 3-2 不同给药剂量的异戊巴比妥钠对小鼠作用的影响

鼠号	体重(g)	药物剂量(mg/kg)	翻正反射消失起效时间(min)	翻正反射消失维持时间(min)
1 号				
2 号				

【注意事项】

(1) 小鼠腹腔注射给药时,针头从下腹部刺入皮下后,再以 45° 斜刺入腹腔,回抽无血液,注射给药。

(2) 穿刺部位不能太高,以防刺入胸腔。

【问题讨论】

不同给药剂量的异戊巴比妥钠对小鼠翻正反射的消失有何影响? 为什么?

(赵蕾)

实验三　不同给药途径对药物作用的影响

一、不同给药途径的异戊巴比妥钠对小鼠的作用

【实验目的】

观察不同给药途径的异戊巴比妥钠对小鼠作用的影响。

【实验原理】

给药途径不同,药物吸收的速度及吸收量不同,直接影响药物的起效时间与效应。相同剂量的异戊巴比妥钠可因给药途径不同而产生不同的作用。

【实验材料】

(1) 器材:钟罩,天平,注射器(1 ml)。

(2) 药品:1% 异戊巴比妥钠溶液。

【实验对象】

昆明系小鼠 4 只，18～22 g/只。

【实验步骤】

（1）取小鼠 4 只，称重并观察正常活动。1、2 号小鼠腹腔注射，3、4 号小鼠灌胃 1% 的异戊巴比妥钠（100 mg/kg），观察小鼠活动情况并记录翻正反射消失的起效时间以及维持时间。

（2）观察项目：翻正反射消失。

（3）请将结果记录于表 3-3。

表 3-3　不同给药途径的异戊巴比妥钠对小鼠作用的影响

鼠号	体重（g）	给药途径	翻正反射消失起效时间（min）	翻正反射消失维持时间（min）
1 号				
2 号				
3 号				
4 号				

【注意事项】

灌胃时将小鼠颈部拉直，自口腔沿上腭轻轻插入灌胃针头，防止液体注入气管。

【问题讨论】

不同给药途径的异戊巴比妥钠对小鼠翻正反射的消失有何影响？为什么？

二、不同给药途径的 $MgSO_4$ 对家兔的作用

【实验目的】

观察不同给药途径的 $MgSO_4$ 对家兔作用的影响。

【实验原理】

$MgSO_4$ 可因给药途径不同而产生不同的药理作用。口服给药后，肠道内的 Mg^{2+} 难以被吸收，导致肠内容物高渗，从而抑制肠内水分的吸收，增加肠腔容积，扩张肠道，刺激肠蠕动，有泻下和利胆的作用。静脉注射 $MgSO_4$ 后，由于 Mg^{2+} 和 Ca^{2+} 化学性质相似，Mg^{2+} 可特异性地与 Ca^{2+} 竞争，拮抗 Ca^{2+} 的作用，从而抑制中枢及外周神经系统依赖 Ca^{2+} 的信号通路，使骨骼肌、心肌、血管平滑肌松弛，从而发挥肌松作用和降压作用。

【实验材料】

（1）器材：兔箱、婴儿秤、注射器（5 ml、10 ml、50 ml）。

（2）药品：5% $MgSO_4$ 溶液，2.5% $CaCl_2$ 溶液。

【实验对象】

新西兰系家兔2只。

【实验步骤】

取家兔2只，称重，观察其正常活动。1号家兔耳缘静脉注射5%的 $MgSO_4$（175 mg/kg），2号家兔灌胃相同剂量的 $MgSO_4$，观察家兔的呼吸、肌张力和大便情况。当家兔出现肌张力下降、呼吸困难等症状，立即给予2.5%的 $CaCl_2$（50 mg/kg）耳缘静脉注射进行解救。将结果记录于表3-4。

表 3-4　不同给药途径的 $MgSO_4$ 对家兔作用的影响

家兔	体重(kg)	给药途径	剂量(mg/kg)	呼吸情况	肌张力	大便
1号						
2号						

【注意事项】

$MgSO_4$ 安全范围窄，过量易引起呼吸抑制、血压骤降和心脏骤停而死亡，故需缓慢静脉注射。

【问题讨论】

不同给药途径的 $MgSO_4$ 对家兔有何不同作用？为什么？

（赵蕾）

实验四　半数有效量(ED_{50})的测定

【实验目的】

（1）观察不同剂量的戊巴比妥钠对小鼠作用的影响。
（2）学习药物半数有效量 ED_{50} 的测定及计算方法。

【实验原理】

药理效应与剂量在一定范围内成比例，这就是剂量-效应关系（dose-effect relationship）。用药物反应的阳性率做纵坐标，对数剂量做横坐标，曲线呈对称的"S"形。曲线在有效率50%处斜率最大，变化最明显。此时剂量也最准确，误差小，通常就把这个剂量称为半数有效量（median effective dose，ED_{50}），即引起半数动物产生阳性反应的剂量。精密测定 ED_{50} 前，通常要摸索合适的剂量范围，即测出能使小鼠出现接近0%及100%阳性反应的剂量。据此进一步选择适当的剂量间比（radio of dose），一般为1：0.8~1：0.7，以确定测定

ED_{50} 的各组剂量。

【实验材料】

（1）器材：钟罩，天平，注射器（1 ml）。
（2）药品：0.245%，0.196%，0.156%，0.125%，0.1% 戊巴比妥钠溶液。

【实验对象】

昆明系小鼠 50 只，18～22 g/只。

【实验材料】

取小鼠 50 只，分为 5 组，每组 10 只，称重并观察正常活动。每组分别腹腔注射不同剂量戊巴比妥钠 49、39、31、25、20 mg/kg，以翻正反射消失作为催眠指标，给药 15 min 内，记录各组出现催眠作用的鼠数。汇集全班结果，将剂量和对应鼠数输入计算机。

表 3-5　测试结果

组别	剂量 D(mg/kg)	实验鼠数	催眠鼠数	催眠反应百分率	ED_{50}(mg/kg)
1	49	10			
2	39	10			
3	31	10			
4	25	10			
5	20	10			

记录计算机中其他参数的值，并分析此药是否安全。

也可用计算公式：$ED_{50} = \log^{-1}[X_m - I(\sum P - 0.5)]$

式中：X_m 为最大剂量对数值；P 为动物阳性率（用小数表示）；I 为相临两组剂量比值的对数（高剂量做分子）；$\sum P$ 为各组阳性率的总和。

【注意事项】

小鼠给药量要准确，随机分组。

【问题分析】

药物的半数有效量、半数致死量、治疗指数及其测定意义。

（赵蕾）

实验五　ABO 血型鉴定

【实验目的】

通过观察红细胞凝集现象，学习 ABO 血型鉴定的原理及测定血型的方法和意义。

【实验原理】

红细胞血型是由红细胞膜表面特异性的抗原决定的。在 ABO 血型系统中,抗原存在于红细胞膜表面,而血清中存在抗体。当 A 抗原与抗 A 抗体相遇或 B 抗原与抗 B 抗体相遇时,将发生特异性红细胞凝集反应。因此,可用已知标准血清中的抗体(A 型标准血清含抗 B 抗体,B 型标准血清含抗 A 抗体)来测定受检者红细胞膜上未知的抗原,根据是否发生红细胞凝集反应来确定血型。

临床上在输血前必须进行血型鉴定,以确保安全输血。

表 3-6　ABO 血型中的抗原和抗体

血型	抗原	抗体
O	无 A 和 B	抗 A 和抗 B
A	A	抗 B
B	B	抗 A
AB	A 和 B	无抗 A 和抗 B

【实验材料】

消毒采血针,双凹玻片,棉球,消毒牙签,培养皿,托盘,显微镜,75%酒精棉球,抗 A 和抗 B 标准血清。

【实验对象】

人。

【实验步骤】

(1) 取干燥清洁双凹玻片 1 片,两端分别标明 A、B 字样。

(2) 在 A 端、B 端凹槽中央分别滴抗 A 标准血清和抗 B 标准血清各 1 滴。

(3) 用 75%酒精棉球消毒采血部位(耳垂或左手无名指指尖),待酒精挥发后,用采血针刺破皮肤,使用过的采血针弃入污物桶。

(4) 捏住消毒牙签中部,用一端取血一滴放入玻片 A 端凹槽中与抗 A 标准血清混合;用另一端取血一滴放入玻片 B 端凹槽中与抗 B 标准血清混合。牙签两端切勿混用。

(5) 室温下放置 1~2 min 后,用肉眼观察有无凝集现象。肉眼不易分辨的用显微镜观察。观察时,注意区别红细胞凝集与红细胞沉积。可水平方向轻轻晃动玻片,红细胞沉积经振摇后呈烟雾状散开,而红细胞凝集则不散开,凝集块越来越大,且血清透亮。

(6) 根据凝集现象判断血型。如果只是 A 端发生凝集,则血型为 A 型;若只是 B 端发生凝集,则为 B 型;若两端均发生凝集,则为 AB 型;若两端均未发生凝集,则为 O 型。

(7) 实验完毕后,清洗用过的玻片,弃掉用过的酒精棉球、采血针、牙签及消毒纸巾。

【注意事项】

（1）采血过程必须严格消毒，以防感染。

（2）采血针要做到一人一针，不能重复使用，更不能混用。

（3）混匀用的牙签两端必须各端专用，且搅拌混匀后不可再取血用，杜绝两种标准血清的混淆。

（4）取血不宜太少以免影响实验结果。

【问题讨论】

（1）根据自己的血型，说明你能接受和输血给何种血型的人，为什么？

（2）已知甲的血型为 A 型，在无标准血清的情况下，能否测出乙的血型？

（石丽娟）

实验六　人体心音听诊

【实验目的】

（1）学习心音听诊的方法。

（2）识别第一心音与第二心音。

【实验原理】

人类的循环系统包括由心脏和血管组成的体循环和肺循环。正常情况下，血液在心血管系统中单向流动。心肌的泵血作用促使血液流动，心脏收缩和舒张时，位于心脏内的 4 个具有单向开放特性的瓣膜开放或关闭。心动周期中，心肌收缩、瓣膜启闭、血液加速度和减速度对心血管壁的加压和减压作用以及形成的涡流等因素引起的机械振动，可通过周围组织传递到胸壁；如将听诊器放在胸壁某些部位，就可以听到声音，称为心音。通过心音听诊，可以了解心脏的健康状况。图 3-3 显示听诊心音的最佳位置。

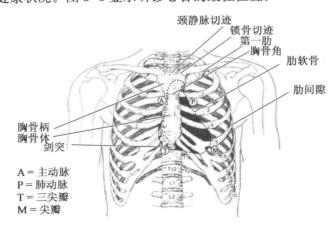

图 3-3　听诊区

38

心音发生在心动周期的某些特定时期,其音调和持续时间也有一定的规律;正常心脏可听到 4 个心音:即第一、第二、第三和第四心音。多数情况下只能听到"咚-嗒"的声音,分别为第一心音和第二心音。第一心音,"咚",发生在心室收缩早期,音调低,持续时间相对较长,在心尖搏动处(左第五肋间与隙锁骨中线交点)听得最清楚。在心室收缩期,房室瓣突然关闭所引起的振动,以及由于心室射血引起大血管扩张及产生的涡流发出的低频振动,是第一心音的主要组成成分。因此,第一心音可以作为心室收缩期开始的标志。第二心音,"嗒",发生在心室舒张期,音调较高,持续时间较短,在胸骨左缘第二肋间听得清楚。其产生主要与主动脉瓣的关闭有关,于标志心室舒张期的开始。

【实验器材】

听诊器。

【实验对象】

人。

【实验步骤】

(1) 受试者安静端坐休息 10 min。

(2) 检查者戴好听诊器,注意听诊器的耳件与外耳道开口方向一致(向前)。

(3) 调整听诊器的位置,找到听诊最清楚的位置。仔细听诊心音,注意区分第一心音和第二心音。

(4) 观察项目:仔细听诊心音,注意区分第一心音和第二心音。如果第一、二心音难以分辨,可用左手触诊心尖搏动或颈动脉脉搏,当手指触及搏动时所听见的心音即为第一心音。

(5) 记录实验结果:心率:___次/分;心律:(齐)。

【注意事项】

(1) 实验室内必须保持安静,以利听诊。

(2) 听诊器耳件应与外耳道方向一致。橡皮管不能交叉,以免发生摩擦音影响听诊。

(3) 如呼吸音影响听诊,可令受试者暂停呼吸片刻。

【问题讨论】

第一心音和第二心音是怎样形成的？它们有何临床意义？

(石丽娟)

实验七　人体动脉血压测定

【实验目的】

(1) 学会间接测量法(听诊法)测定人体动脉血压。

（2）了解动脉血压的正常值。

【实验原理】

在一个心动周期内,动脉血压是发生变化的。心室收缩推动血液快速进入动脉,导致动脉血压急剧升高,血液向外周流动,心室舒张,血压逐渐降低直至下一次收缩之前。心室收缩血压升到最高值(收缩压),心室舒张血压降到最低值(舒张压)。可以通过在动脉插入导管记录收缩压和舒张压,这种直接测量的方法比较准确,但是对机体是有创伤的,并且不方便。而间接测量血压的方法因对机体基本没有创伤,且操作简单,更容易被接受。

临床上测量人体动脉血压最常用的方法是间接测量上臂肱动脉的血压。即用血压计的袖带在肱动脉外加压,根据血管音的变化来测量血压。通常血液在血管内连续流动时没有声音。当将空气打入缠绕于上臂的袖带内,使其压力超过收缩压时,便可完全阻断肱动脉内的血流,此时,用听诊器在其远端听不到声音,如缓慢放气以逐渐降低袖带内压力,当外加压力稍低于肱动脉收缩压而高于舒张压时,血液可断续流过被压血管,形成涡流而发出声音。所听到的第一声时的外加压力作为收缩压值。继续放气,当袖带内压力刚低于舒张压时,血管内的血流由断续变为连续,声音突然由强变弱或消失,此时的外加压力作为舒张压值。

【实验器材】

血压计,听诊器。

【实验对象】

人。

【实验步骤】

（1）受试者脱去一侧手臂衣袖,全身放松静坐 5 min。
（2）受检者前臂平放在桌上,掌心向上,使上臂中心部与心脏位置同高。
（3）血压计袖带绑于受试者上臂,其下缘应在肘关节上 1～2 cm 处。
（4）在肘窝内侧扪到肱动脉脉搏后,将听诊器的听筒放于肱动脉搏动处(图3-4)。
（5）观察项目:打开血压计,给袖带加压至听不到脉搏音为止;慢慢放气降低袖带压力(1～2 mmHg/s),在观察水银柱缓缓下降的同时仔细听诊;在听到"崩"样第一声清晰而短促脉搏音时,血压表上所示水银柱高度即代表收缩压。继续缓慢降低袖带压力,声音突然由强变弱(或声音变调)这一瞬间,血压表上所示水银柱高度代表舒张压。也有人把声音突然消失时血压计上所示水银柱高度作为舒张压;记录你所测得同学的血压:收缩压/舒张压 mmHg(kPa)。

【注意事项】

（1）实验室内必须保持安静,以利听诊。
（2）听诊器耳件应与外耳道方向一致。橡皮管不能交叉,以免发生摩擦音影响听诊。
（3）测量血压前需嘱受试者静坐放松,以排除体力活动及精神紧张对血压的影响。
（4）袖带缠绕不能太紧或太松。

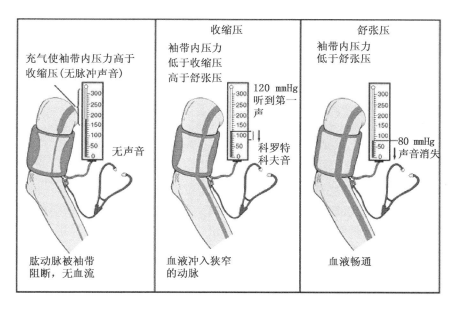

图 3-4 血压测定

（5）发现血压超过正常范围时，应将袖带解下，让受试者休息 10 min 后再测。

（6）实验结束后，一定要关闭血压计开关。

【问题讨论】

（1）哪些因素可影响动脉血压的测定？

（2）测动脉血压时，放气速度为何不宜太快或太慢？

（石丽娟）

实验八　药物血浆半衰期测定

【实验目的】

1. 学习用比色法测定水杨酸的血浆药物浓度。

2. 掌握药物血浆半衰期的计算方法。

【实验原理】

大多数药物在体内按一级动力学的规律消除。当药物分布相完成后，以血浆药物浓度的对数值为纵座标，时间为横座标，药-时曲线在半对数坐标图上作图时呈为直线。根据药后消除相各时间点测出的血浆药物浓度与时间进行直线回归，可得到直线方程：$Ct = \log C_0 - k/2.303\, t$。从该方程可算出血药浓度下降一半所需时间，即药物血浆浓度半衰期（plasma half-life，$t_{1/2}$），其计算公式为 $t_{1/2} = 0.693/k$。

【实验材料】

器材：手术器械一套，兔台，动脉插管，动脉夹，试管架，试管，微量移液器，注射器，分光光度计,离心机,计算机。

药品:25%乌拉坦,10%水杨酸钠,10%三氯醋酸,10%三氯化铁,1%肝素。

【实验对象】

家兔。

【实验步骤】

1. 颈总动脉插管手术

取家兔一只,称重后耳缘静脉缓慢注射25%乌拉坦(4 ml/kg, 1 g/kg)。麻醉后背位固定于兔台上,剪毛,切开皮肤,分离皮下组织,暴露一侧颈总动脉。远心端用棉线结扎,近心端用动脉夹夹闭。耳缘静脉注入1%的肝素1 ml/kg实施全身肝素化抗凝。用眼科剪在远心端处剪一切口,向心脏方向插入已局部肝素化的颈动脉插管,用棉线结扎固定,以备后续采集血样用。

2. 血液样本采集和给药

打开动脉夹,采集药前的血液样本放入试管内,采集量≥1 ml。由耳缘静脉注入10%水杨酸钠(1.5 ml/kg, 150 mg/kg),注射完毕记录时间。分别于给药后5、15、25、35、45 min从颈总动脉采集≥1 ml血液样本。

3. 血药浓度测定

(1)方法一

准确取1 ml血样,置于相应标记的试管中,每管分别加入10%三氯醋酸3.5 ml,充分摇匀后离心(2 000~2 500转/分,5分钟)。准确吸取每管上清液3 ml,分别转移至做好相应标记的试管中,每管分别加入10%三氯化铁0.3 ml摇匀,显色。用分光光度计测定各管在波长520 nm处的光密度,以药前管做对照,校正零点。

(2)方法二

准确取1 ml血样,置于相应标记的试管中,每管分别加入10%三氯醋酸3.5 ml,充分摇匀后离心(2 000~2 500转/分,5分钟)。准确吸取每管上清液3 ml,分别转移至做好相应标记的试管中,用分光光度计测定各管在波长300 nm处的光密度,以药前管做对照,校正零点。

实验结果填入表3-7。

表3-7 水杨酸钠的时间-光密度数据

时间(min)	用药前	用药后				
		5	15	25	30	45
光密度						

4. 半衰期计算

(1)采用RM6240 EC多道生理信号采集处理系统计算。选择药理学实验,$t_{1/2}$计算。再分别输入药后时间和对应的光密度值,当数据输入完成后,按"计算"即可得到水杨酸钠的血浆半衰期及消除速率方程。

(2)根据公式计算水杨酸钠的血浆半衰期。

42

$$t_{1/2} = 0.301(t_2 - t_1)/\lg D_1 - \lg D_2$$

t_1、t_2为药后采血时间点,D_1、D_2分别为相对应的光密度值。

【注意事项】

1. 静脉给药时避免将药物误入皮下。
2. 每次取样必须准确,否则会影响最后的结果。

【问题讨论】

1. 测定药物血浆半衰期有何临床意义?
2. 一级动力学消除有哪些特点?

(刘桦)

实验九　有机磷农药中毒及解救

【实验目的】

观察有机磷农药中毒的症状及阿托品、碘解磷定对有机磷农药中毒的解救效果,初步分析其解救原理。

【实验原理】

有机磷农药能与胆碱酯酶牢固结合,使之失去水解乙酰胆碱(Ach)的活性,造成突触间隙 Ach 大量堆积而产生一系列中毒症状(M 样、N 样症状等)。阿托品是 M 受体阻断药,碘解磷定是胆碱酯酶复活药,可不同程度地解救其中毒症状。如阿托品解除 M 样症状,但对肌震颤无效;碘解磷定可使胆碱酯酶复活,对肌震颤有效。

【实验材料】

(1) 器材:兔箱、注射器(1、5、10 ml)、尺子、滤纸。
(2) 药品:5%敌百虫、0.05%阿托品、2.5%碘解磷定。

【实验对象】

家兔。

【实验步骤】

(1) 家兔 1 只,称重,观察各项指标:活动情况、呼吸、瞳孔大小、唾液、大小便及有无肌震颤等,分别记录。

(2) 给家兔耳缘静脉注射 5%敌百虫 75 mg/kg,观察上述各项指标(一般在给药后10～15 min内出现症状),并加以记录。待中毒症状明显时,立即耳缘静脉注射 0.05%阿托品 1 mg/kg(2 ml/kg),观察症状有何改善,在症状明显改善后(约 10 min),再静注 2.5%碘解磷定 75 mg/kg(3 ml/kg),观察中毒症状消除情况并记录。

43

【观察项目】

（1）呼吸：有无呼吸困难。

（2）瞳孔：用尺子量出左右两侧瞳孔的直径，以 mm 表示其大小，测定时注意光线强弱要相同。

（3）唾液：用滤纸按吸嘴部，看纸上水迹大小以无唾液（－）、有唾液（＋）、唾液较多（＋＋）、唾液很多（＋＋＋）表示。

（4）大小便：按量的多少以无大小便（－）、有大便和/或小便（＋）、大便和/或小便较多（＋＋）、大便和/或小便很多以至腹部毛都湿透（＋＋＋）表示。

（5）肌震颤：按程度不同以无肌震颤（－）、局部或间有肌震颤（＋）、全身肌震颤（＋＋）、全身肌震颤并站立不稳或由兴奋转入抑制，瘫卧桌上（＋＋＋）表示。

表 3-8　有机磷农药中毒及药物解救后症状

药　　物	呼吸状况	瞳孔大小	唾液分泌	大小便	肌震颤
用药前					
敌百虫					
阿托品					
碘解磷定					

【注意事项】

（1）敌百虫为剧毒药，可从皮肤吸收，如不慎接触后应立即清水冲洗，切勿用肥皂，因其在碱性环境中可转变为毒性更大的敌敌畏。

（2）瞳孔的大小是受光照的影响，整个实验过程中光条件应保持一致。

（3）注意观察症状并及时记录。

【问题讨论】

（1）有机磷农药中毒的机制是什么？

（2）阿托品及碘解磷定解救有机磷农药中毒的机制是什么，它们的解救原理有何不同？

（孙玲美）

实验十　巴比妥类药物的抗惊厥作用

【实验目的】

掌握电刺激诱导惊厥的方法，观察巴比妥类药物的抗惊厥作用。

【实验原理】

巴比妥类药物对中枢神经系统有普遍性抑制作用，其随着剂量的增加，其对中枢抑制的作用由弱变强，相应表现为镇静、催眠、抗惊厥及抗癫痫、麻醉等作用。

【实验材料】

（1）器材：药理生理多用仪，钟罩，滴管，注射器，腭鱼夹，天平。

（2）药品：0.5%苯巴比妥钠，生理盐水。

【实验对象】

雄性昆明系小鼠 2 只，体重 18～22 g/只。

【实验步骤】

1. 药理生理多用仪参数设定

多用仪正面：刺激方式设为单次，时间设为 0.25 s，频率可在 8～1 Hz 之间进行调节。

多用仪背面：选择开关拨向电惊厥激怒一端，电压调至 90 V，交流输出端接上腭鱼夹备用。

2. 惊厥实验

取小鼠 2 只，秤重，编号。将多用仪交流输出端的两只腭鱼夹一只夹在小鼠两耳间的皮肤上，另一只夹在下颌的皮肤上，接通电源，按下多用仪正面的启动按钮，即可输出一次电刺激。固定电压，调节频率，确定可使两只小鼠产生电惊厥的频率。实验中注意观察小鼠产生电惊厥的过程：僵直屈曲期——后肢伸直期——阵挛期——恢复期。本实验以小鼠后肢伸直作为产生电惊厥的指标。然后一只小鼠腹腔注射 0.5%苯巴比妥钠（50 mg/kg），另一只腹腔注射相应剂量的生理盐水作对照。给药 30 min 后，分别以给药前各自的电惊厥频率进行刺激，观察两鼠有何不同反应？

3. 实验结果

将实验结果填入表 3-9。

表 3-9　药物对抗小鼠电惊厥作用

动物号	体重（g）	药物	剂量（mg/kg）	阈值频率（Hz）	后肢伸直	
					药前	药后
1						
2						

【注意事项】

（1）由于动物个体差异，电惊厥频率而有所不同，调节时频率应由大到小。

（2）用药前后注意采用相同的电惊厥频率刺激。

（3）多用仪背面选择开关在实验过程中始终拨向电惊厥激怒一端。

【问题讨论】

巴比妥类药物的抗惊厥作用机制是什么？

（朱新建）

实验十一　氯丙嗪对小鼠激怒反应的影响

【实验目的】

掌握电刺激诱导小鼠激怒反应的方法，观察氯丙嗪的安定作用。

【实验原理】

氯丙嗪对中枢神经系统有较强的抑制作用，能显著控制动物的活动状态和躁狂状态，减少动物的攻击行为，也称神经安定作用。

【实验材料】

（1）器材：药理生理多用仪，钟罩，电激怒盒，注射器，烧杯，天平。
（2）药品：0.05%氯丙嗪，生理盐水。

【实验对象】

雄性昆明系小鼠 4 只，体重 18～22 g/只。

【实验步骤】

1. 药理生理多用仪参数设定
多用仪正面：刺激方式设定为连续，时间设定为 1 s，频率为 8 Hz。
多用仪背面：选择开关拨向电惊厥激怒一端，电压在 60～90 V 之间调节，交流输出端接上电激怒盒备用。

2. 激怒反应实验
取异笼饲养小鼠 4 只，秤重编号。随机取两只小鼠放于电激怒盒的铜丝板上，用钟罩将其罩住。接通多用仪电源开关，交流输出端即可输出连续电刺激。调节电压大小，找出能使两只小鼠出现激怒反应的最小电压。以两只小鼠两前肢离地直立，相互对峙，互相撕咬，作为小鼠出现激怒反应的观察指标。激怒反应的电压阈值确定后，然后一对小鼠腹腔注射 0.05%氯丙嗪（5 mg/kg），另一对小鼠腹腔注射相应剂量的生理盐水作为对照。给药 30 min 后以分别以给药前各自的电压阈值电刺激，观察两组小鼠给药前后有何不同反应。

3. 实验数据
将实验结果填入表 3-10。

表 3-10　氯丙嗪对小鼠激怒反应的影响

动物号	体　重（g）	药物	剂量（mg/kg）	阈值电压（V）	激怒反应	
					药前	药后
1						
2						
3						
4						

（1）由于动物个体差异，激怒反应的电压阈值有所不同，调节时电压应由小到大。
（2）用药前后注意采用相同的电压阈值刺激。
（3）多用仪背面选择开关在实验过程中始终拨向电惊厥激怒一端。

【问题讨论】

氯丙嗪的安定作用机制是什么？

（朱新建）

实验十二　神经干动作电位的记录与观察

【实验目的】

（1）制备蟾蜍坐骨神经干标本，记录电刺激引起的神经干复合动作电位。
（2）观察坐骨神经干双相动作电位、单相动作电位的基本波形，分析其产生原理。
（3）分析刺激参数对坐骨神经干动作电位的影响及其机制。
（4）学习测定神经干动作电位传导速度的方法并了解其原理。

【实验原理】

可兴奋细胞受到有效刺激后，膜电位将产生一次快速的、可向远端传播的电位波动，此即为动作电位（action potential，AP）。神经的动作电位是神经兴奋的客观标志。

神经纤维受到阈刺激或阈上刺激而产生 AP 时，兴奋部位的细胞膜表面相对于未兴奋部位呈负电位；AP 将以局部电流的形式进行双向传导。如果两个引导电极置于兴奋性正常的神经干外表面，借助于生物信号采集分析系统，用引导电极可引导出神经冲动先后通过两个电极处而产生的两个方向相反的电位波形，称为双相动作电位（图3-5）。如果两个引导电极之间的神经纤维完全损伤，神经冲动只通过第一个引导电极，不能传至第二个引导电极，则只能引导出一个方向的电位偏转波形，称为单相动作电位。

单根神经纤维受刺激而产生的动作电位遵循"全或无"规律。神经干由许多不同类型的神经纤维组成，神经干动作电位是由许多神经纤维动作电位叠加而成的综合性电位变化，是一种复合动作电位。神经干动作电位幅度在一定范围内可随刺激强度的增大而增高。

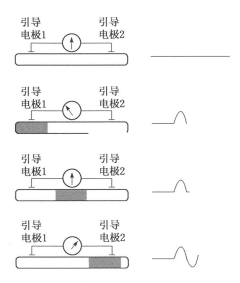

图 3-5　双向动作电位的记录原理

动作电位在神经干上传导具有一定的速度（v）。测定神经冲动在神经干上传导的距离

（d）与通过这段距离所需的时间（t），可根据 $v = d / t$ 求出神经冲动的传导速度。

【实验材料】

（1）器材：RM6240 EC 多道生理信号采集处理系统，蛙板，蛙钉，250 ml 烧杯，培养皿，污物碗，探针，组织剪，眼科剪，眼科镊，有齿镊，丝线，玻璃分针，纱布，神经屏蔽盒。

（2）药品：任氏液。

【实验对象】

蟾蜍。

【实验步骤】

1. 制备蟾蜍坐骨神经干标本

（1）捣毁脑脊髓：取蟾蜍一只，用自来水冲洗干净，左手握住蟾蜍，用食指压其头部前端、拇指按压其背部，使头前俯。右手持探针由枕骨大孔垂直刺入，将探针向前伸入颅腔，左右搅动捣毁脑组织；再将探针抽回至枕骨大孔，向尾端刺入椎管、搅动捣毁脊髓。脑和脊髓完全破坏后，可见动物四肢松软。

（2）剪除躯干上部及内脏：左手拇指及食指于骶髂关节上缘夹持蟾蜍脊柱尾侧，其余 3 指将蟾蜍双后肢收拔于手心；右手持组织剪，在蟾蜍骶髂关节水平上 0.5～1 cm 处横断脊柱，然后沿躯干两侧剪开腹部皮肤、剪除躯干上部及内脏。

（3）剥去后肢皮肤：左手持有齿镊，夹持脊柱断端（注意勿触碰坐骨神经），右手捏住其旁皮肤边缘，剥除全部后肢皮肤。将标本放入盛有任氏液的烧杯中。

（4）清洗双手及使用过的探针、剪刀等器械后，再进行下述步骤。

（5）分离两后肢：用有齿镊从背位夹住脊柱将标本由任氏液中提出，剪去尾骨（注意勿损伤坐骨神经），然后用剪刀沿脊柱正中线及耻骨联合中央剪开，双后肢即完全分离。将标本浸入烧杯任氏液中。

（6）制备坐骨神经干标本：用蛙钉将标本仰卧位固定于蛙板上，用玻璃分针沿脊柱旁侧游离坐骨神经，靠近中枢端穿线、结扎。再将标本俯位固定，剪断梨状肌及其附近结缔组织；用玻璃分针循股二头肌和半膜肌之间的坐骨神经沟，纵向分离暴露坐骨神经，用玻璃分针小心游离、经过腘窝至腓神经跟腱端。在暴露好的坐骨神经（腓神经）跟腱端穿线、结扎，在结扎点远端剪断神经。利用结扎线轻轻提起神经，辨清坐骨神经走向，置眼科剪于神经干与周围组织之间，由外周端向中枢端小心剪断神经干沿途分支（不可撕扯），直至脊柱旁的前一结扎点，在此结扎线中枢端、剪断神经干。分离出的坐骨神经标本浸入盛有任氏液的培养皿中待用。

2. 连接系统，选择实验模块

（1）连接生物信号采集处理系统与神经屏蔽盒。

（2）启动 RM 6240 EC 多道生理信号采集处理系统，进入"神经干传导速度的测定"实验模块。此模块中仪器参数基本设置为：

时间常数：0.001 s；滤波频率：1 kHz；

采样频率：40 kHz；灵敏度：2 mV；扫描速度：0.5～1 ms/div；

强度递增刺激模式:同步触发;刺激强度:0.1～3 V;刺激波宽:0.1 ms;强度增量:0.01 V;延迟:5 ms。

3. 信号采集及观察

(1) 用任氏液棉球擦拭神经屏蔽盒的所有电极。将一任氏液浸湿的丝线搭置于刺激电极和引导电极上,开始刺激及采样。观察显示器波形,判断系统连接状态、信号采集处理效果,以及有无干扰。若信号正常(扫描光滑、无干扰信号,可有刺激伪迹),即可停止采样,去掉丝线。

(2) 小心将浸于培养皿任氏液中的坐骨神经干标本提起,将其搭置于屏蔽盒内电极上,令其中枢端朝向刺激电极、外周端朝向引导电极,并确保神经干与各电极均接触良好。盖好屏蔽盒,即可开始实验观察。

【观察项目】

(1) 给标本以电刺激(在一定刺激波宽下,由小及大逐渐增大刺激强度),观察所记录到的电位波形。辨识刺激伪迹与神经干双相动作电位。

(2) 分析刺激强度与双相动作电位幅值的关系。在一定刺激波宽条件下(如 0.2 ms),选择"强度递增刺激",观察随刺激强度增大、双相动作电位波幅的改变,记录最大刺激强度(即在一定刺激波宽条件下,动作电位幅值不再随刺激强度增大而增加时的临界刺激强度)。

(3) 测量最大刺激强度下神经干双相动作电位的潜伏期;动作电位第一相和第二相的波幅与波宽,分析双相动作电位是否为对称波形。

(4) 分析刺激波的波宽与阈强度的关系。记录 3 组不同刺激波宽时的阈强度(即在某一刺激波宽条件下刚刚出现双相动作电位时的临界刺激强度)。

(5) 测量神经干动作电位传导速度。给予神经干适当刺激,观察两对引导电极分别引导到的双相动作电位波形。测量两路双相动作电位起始点(或第一相波的波峰顶点)之间的时间差值 t;测量屏蔽盒内两对引导电极之间的距离 d;计算神经干动作电位的传导速度 v($v = d/t$)(图 3-6)。

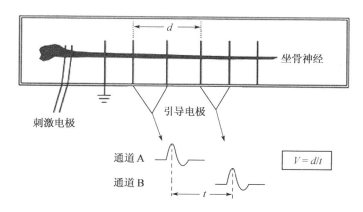

图 3-6 测量神经干动作电位传导速度

(6) 单相动作电位的观察。用镊子将第二对引导电极之间的神经夹伤,再次给予电刺激,观察两路动作电位波形。可见第二路动作电位由原来的双相变为单相。

【注意事项】

（1）坐骨神经干标本制备要仔细、轻柔,避免损伤。

（2）坐骨神经干标本制备以及实验过程中,均应注意保持其活性良好,经常用任氏液湿润之。

（3）屏蔽盒内电极间不能积存水滴,以防短路。

【问题讨论】

（1）如果以湿棉线代替神经干标本,会记录到什么结果?

（2）实验中怎样辨别刺激伪迹与动作电位?

（3）单根神经纤维的动作电位与神经干的复合动作电位有哪些不同?

（刘莉洁）

实验十三　水肿发生因素的分析

【实验目的】

通过一定的实验模型探讨毛细血管内压、胶体渗透压等因素在水肿形成中的意义。

【实验原理】

利用蟾蜍循环系统,从主动脉弓定量灌入一定性质的液体,同时收集主要从肝静脉灌出的液体,比较灌出液与灌入液两者"量"的差异,推断体内是否存在液体潴留。

【实验材料】

（1）器材:手术器械1套,血管灌流装置1套,10 ml量筒2只,50 ml烧杯2只,25 ml烧杯1只,滴管1只,1 ml注射器1只。

（2）药品:1%肝素,任氏液,低分子右旋糖酐溶液。

【实验对象】

蟾蜍。

【实验步骤】

1. 蟾蜍血管灌流装置的准备

将20 ml注射器空筒与一段带有止水夹的输液器导管相连,导管另一端与插有细塑料管的针柄相连。再将注射器空筒固定于铁支台试管夹上,于距离注射器空筒乳头部30 cm处在铁支台上安一双凹夹,再以此固定一烧瓶夹,用以固定蛙板。通过输液器导管上的止水夹调节滴流速度。然后用任氏液驱尽气泡,充满整个灌流系统。关闭止水夹待用。

2. 动物处理

用金属探针捣毁蟾蜍的脑、脊髓,仰位放置在蛙板上。用剪刀沿腹正中线偏左约

0.5 cm剖开腹腔,向腹壁静脉内注入1%肝素0.1 ml,然后向上剖开胸腔,剪开胸锁联合关节,沿肩胛骨向两侧剪至脊柱旁。再将腹部切口下缘向两侧剪开,使灌出液不会积滞在体腔凹陷处。最后用眼科剪剪开心包膜,暴露心脏。

3. 蟾蜍血管灌流实验

翻转肝脏,暴露后腔静脉,于其后方穿一根线留待之后用以阻断部分静脉回流。再于一侧主动脉弓后穿2根线,结扎近心端(留线头用做牵引),旋即用眼科剪在贴近该结扎线根部远心侧的主动脉上斜剪一小口,将充满任氏液的细塑料管向远心端插入并结扎固定。剪开一侧肝静脉,以利灌流液外流,同时将此蛙板倾斜安放在上面准备的血管灌流装置中,调节止水夹,将灌流速度调至25~30滴/min左右,然后进行以下实验。

(1)以小量筒量取10 ml任氏液,当注射器空筒内灌入液面降至基线(注射器空筒乳头部的标线)时立即倒入筒内,同时用一小烧杯承接自蛙板一角滴下的水滴。本实验系通过对比灌出液与灌入液量之差别来判断是否有液体在体内积滞,故务必做到倾注灌入液与承接灌出液同时开始,并避免灌出液积滞于体腔或流失。应注意注射器空筒内灌入液液面,当其降至基线时重新倾注10 ml任氏液至筒内,并立即撤换小烧杯,记录收集到的灌出液量,此即为灌入10 ml任氏液的流出量。并重复一次实验。

(2)向注射器空筒内加入低分子右旋糖酐溶液10 ml,并以小烧杯承接灌出液直到灌入液降至基线,记录流出量。并重复一次实验。

(3)向注射器空筒加入任氏液10 ml后立即结扎后腔静脉,以小烧杯承接灌出液,直至灌入液降至基线,记录流出量。并重复一次实验。

4. 实验数据

将各次灌流结果填入表3-11,比较3种不同条件下灌出液与灌入液在量上的差别。

表3-11 不同因素对蟾蜍血管灌流结果的影响

施加因素		灌入液(ml)	灌出液(ml)
任氏液	第一次	10	
	第二次	10	
右旋糖酐液	第一次	10	
	第二次	10	
任氏液＋静脉结扎	第一次	10	
	第二次	10	

【注意事项】

(1)彻底暴露蟾蜍胸、腹腔,以使灌出液不至积滞在体腔凹陷处。

(2)在注射器空筒乳头部系一根线作为基线,让该基线距离蛙板30 cm。每次灌入液液面下降至此高度时再加入一定量液体。注意将蛙板向一边倾斜,使灌出液朝一个方向流淌。

(3)用任氏液驱尽灌流管道中的气泡,以免形成气栓。

(4)血管内肝素化可保持灌流持续通畅。

(5)分离出主动脉弓后,先结扎其近心端,结扎线头不剪断留作牵引。远心端再穿一根线。在近心端结扎线根部的远侧方向血管部位剪一小口,向远心端插管,注意避免将动脉插破。

(6) 因不同灌注液黏滞度不同,流速也不尽相同,应及时调整灌入速度。

(7) 量取各种灌入液前必须用清水洗净量筒,务必提前准确量取灌入液。

【问题分析】

(1) 灌入任氏液后,灌出液的量有何变化? 为什么出现该变化?

(2) 灌入低分子右旋糖酐溶液后,灌出液的量有何变化? 为什么出现该变化?

(3) 同时灌入任氏液与结扎后腔静脉后,灌出液的量有何变化? 为什么出现该变化?

(廖凯 余卫平)

实验十四 缺 氧

【实验目的】

(1) 了解缺氧类型,制备低张性缺氧与血液性缺氧动物模型。

(2) 观察不同类型缺氧动物模型呼吸和血液颜色变化情况,并分析相关机制。

【实验原理】

(1) 通过窒息制备低张性缺氧模型。

(2) 通过 CO 中毒、亚硝酸盐中毒制备血液性缺氧模型。

【实验材料】

(1) 器材:3 个 500 ml 带塞广口瓶,2 个 125 ml 广口瓶,两支滴管,3 支 1 ml 注射器,1 张双凹玻片,1 把剪刀。

(2) 药品:0.5% 美兰,1% $NaNO_2$ 溶液,10% $NaOH$ 溶液,CO 气囊。

【实验对象】

小鼠。

【实验步骤】

1. 低张性缺氧

(1) 取体重相近的 2 只小鼠,分别放入不加塞的 125 ml 广口瓶内,观察小鼠的正常情况、呼吸频率(次/10 s× 6)与口唇、耳、尾等皮肤颜色。

(2) 塞紧其中一个装鼠瓶的瓶塞,使之密闭并计时,另一只装鼠瓶不加塞作为对照,每隔 3 min 观察上述指标一次。

(3) 记录加塞瓶中小鼠死亡时间。用脊髓离断术处死对照鼠。解剖两鼠,对比内脏颜色,并留待全部实验结束后与其他模型小鼠对比内脏颜色。

（4）对照鼠心脏取血作 CO 定性试验。

2. 血液性缺氧

（1）CO 中毒

① 取 3 只小鼠，分别置于 3 个 500 ml 广口瓶中，将瓶标号为(1)、(2)、(3)。观察小鼠的正常情况、呼吸频率(次/10 s× 6)与口唇、耳、尾等皮肤颜色。

② 于瓶(1)、瓶(2)内分别注入 15 ml CO 后立即塞紧瓶塞，同时将瓶(3)塞紧作对照。计时。

③ 观察小鼠上述指标变化，若发现瓶(1)或瓶(2)内有一小鼠发生抽搐，立即取出，置通风处，观察其变化。让另一小鼠中毒死亡，计时并进行解剖，观察其血液和内脏颜色。从心脏取血做 CO 定性实验。对照鼠及时取出。

附：CO 定性试验(NaOH 法)：于双凹玻片的凹槽内各滴入 2 滴 10% NaOH，然后从 CO 中毒鼠或对照鼠取血一滴分别加入一侧凹槽内，与其中 NaOH 溶液混合反应。含 CO 血能保持粉红色数分钟，而不含 CO 血立即变成棕色。

（2）亚硝酸盐中毒

① 取体重相近的两只小鼠，观察其一般情况与口唇、耳、尾颜色及呼吸频率。

② 取一小鼠腹腔注入 1% $NaNO_2$ 溶液 1 ml，每隔 2 min 计数呼吸频率一次，并观察一般情况及耳、唇、尾颜色，直至小鼠死亡。然后解剖，观察血液与内脏颜色。

③ 取另一小鼠腹腔注入 1% $NaNO_2$ 溶液 1 ml，5 min 后注入 0.5% 美兰 0.4 ml，继续观察直至小鼠恢复或死亡。

附：美兰(MB)解毒机制：

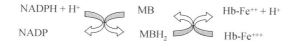

$$NADPH + H^+ \qquad MB \qquad Hb\text{-}Fe^{++} + H^+$$
$$NADP \qquad MBH_2 \qquad Hb\text{-}Fe^{+++}$$

【观察项目】

观察以下项目并完成表 3-12。

表 3-12 各缺氧模型鼠观察结果记录

缺氧模型	呼吸(次/min)	黏膜、皮肤颜色	血液颜色	内脏颜色
对照鼠				
窒息鼠				
CO 中毒鼠				
$NaNO_2$ 中毒鼠				

（1）呼吸频率(次/10 s × 6)；

（2）口唇、耳、尾等黏膜、皮肤颜色；

（3）实验小鼠抽搐；

（4）实验小鼠死亡时间；

（5）血液颜色；

（6）内脏颜色。

【注意事项】

（1）制备低张性缺氧模型时瓶塞要塞紧。

（2）注射器勿混用。应注意药物用量。

（3）应注意各小鼠标号，抢救动物应及时。

（4）取 CO 中毒鼠与对照鼠的血同时做 CO 定性实验。

【问题分析】

（1）低张性缺氧与血液性缺氧时，皮肤、黏膜会是怎样的颜色？

（2）根据本实验结果，各型缺氧时呼吸与组织颜色变化的机制有哪些？

（3）什么是发绀？哪些类型缺氧可有发绀？

（廖凯　余卫平）

实验十五　呼吸运动的调节

【实验目的】

（1）观察影响呼吸运动的各种因素，并分析其作用机制。

（2）学习记录呼吸运动的方法。

【实验原理】

呼吸运动是由呼吸肌的节律性收缩活动所引起的胸廓的扩大和缩小，是肺通气的动力来源，也是整个呼吸过程的基础，其节律性起源于呼吸中枢。呼吸运动的频率和深度会随着机体内、外环境的改变而发生相应的变化，以适应机体代谢活动对气体（O_2 和 CO_2）交换的需要。呼吸运动所发生的适应性的变化有赖于神经系统的反射性调节。其中较为重要的有呼吸中枢、化学感受性的反射、肺牵张反射（肺扩张反射和肺萎陷反射），呼吸肌本体感受性反射等。因此，体内外相关的各种刺激，可以直接作用于中枢部位或通过不同的感受器反射性地影响呼吸运动。

【实验材料】

（1）器材：RM6240 EC 多道生理信号采集处理系统，哺乳动物手术器械 1 套，兔手术操作台，张力传感器，气管插管，玻璃分针，注射器 20 ml 2 个，5 ml 1 个，头皮针，30 cm 橡皮管，纱布 4 块，绑腿绳 4 根，绑牙绳 1 根，粗棉线，细丝线，CO_2 气囊，小钩子。

（2）药品：25% 乌拉坦，3% 乳酸，生理盐水，CO_2 气体。

【实验对象】

家兔。

【实验步骤】

（1）抓兔，称重，从兔耳缘静脉注射 25% 乌拉坦（4 ml/kg，1 g/kg）进行麻醉。待麻醉后仰卧位固定于操作台上,前肢固定为水平位或斜下位。

(2)颈部手术:剪去颈前部被毛,在甲状软骨下方约2 cm处沿颈部正中线切开皮肤,以此点为中心向上下切开约5～7 cm的手术切口。用止血钳钝性分离颈前部的肌肉,暴露气管,把甲状软骨以下的气管与周围组织分离,在气管下放置一棉线备用。在甲状腺下面约第5～7个软骨环上做一倒"T"形切口(如图3-7),插入气管插管,用备用的粗棉线固定。分离气管两侧的迷走神经,各穿一根细丝线备用。手术完毕后用生理盐水纱布覆盖手术伤口部位。

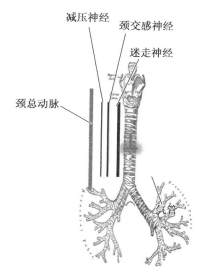

图3-7　颈总动脉鞘内结构及气管
倒"T"形切口示意图

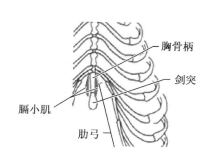

图3-8　膈小肌示意图

(3)上腹部手术:剪去上腹部的毛,确定手术部位。首先找到剑突,在剑突正前方处切开皮肤约2 cm。沿腹白线开腹,切口约2 cm,暴露剑突,游离剑突周围的腹膜,用蚊式钳将膈小肌(如图3-8)与胸骨分离,剪断胸骨,用止血钳锁住近心端。在剑突正中穿带线的小钩子,修剪剑突呈倒三角形。

(4)连接系统,选择实验模块

① 将张力换能器与膈小肌小钩连接,张力换能器则连线RM6240 EC多道生理信号采集处理系统。

② 启动RM6240 EC多道生理信号采集处理系统,进入"呼吸运动调节"实验模块。连接示意图(如图3-9)。

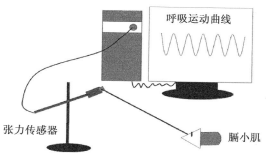

图3-9　生物信号采集处理系统
与膈小肌连接示意图

【观察项目】

(1)观察家兔的正常呼吸曲线,区分吸气相和呼气相。

（2）将气管插管一侧夹闭，使家兔吸入高浓度 CO_2，观察呼吸运动的变化。分析其作用机制。

（3）待呼吸恢复正常，仍将气管插管一侧夹闭，另一侧连接一长 30 cm 橡胶管，观察呼吸运动的变化。分析其作用机制。

（4）待呼吸恢复正常，仍将气管插管一侧夹闭，另一侧夹闭气管插管口径的 1/2～2/3，观察呼吸运动的变化。分析其作用机制。

（5）待呼吸恢复正常，不夹闭气管插管，耳缘静脉注射 3% 乳酸（1 ml/kg），观察呼吸运动的变化。分析其作用机制。

（6）观察牵张反射：

① 待呼吸恢复正常，在家兔吸气末向其肺内注射 20 ml 空气，然后停留 5～10 s，观察呼吸运动的变化。分析其原因。

② 待呼吸恢复正常，在呼气末从肺内抽出 20 ml 气体，然后停留 5～10 s，观察呼吸运动的变化。分析其原因。

（7）剪断双侧迷走神经，观察家兔呼吸运动的变化。分析其原因。

（8）重复步骤 6 的操作，观察呼吸运动的变化。分析其原因。

（9）实验结束后存盘。

（10）实验结果填入表 3-13。

表 3-13　不同因素对呼吸频率与振幅的影响

项　　目		频率（次/min）	振幅（cm）
正常对照		正常	正常
CO_2			
无效腔			
气道阻力			
乳酸			
肺牵张反射	肺扩张反射		
	肺萎陷反射		
切断双侧迷走神经			
切断双侧迷走神经	肺扩张反射		
	肺萎陷反射		

【注意事项】

（1）膈小肌分离时，用蚊式钳进行分离，尽可能减小对膈小肌的损伤；游离剑突时避免形成气胸。

（2）当膈小肌与换能器连接时，连接线与换能器的平面垂直，力量不分散，记录数据较准确。当记录呼吸运动曲线时，避免移动家兔或连接线。

（3）上腹部切口不宜过大，约为 2 cm，避免腹腔脏器触碰膈小肌。

【问题讨论】

（1）根据实验结果，分析高浓度的 CO_2、乳酸和增加无效腔这 3 种因素中那种对呼吸运动作用最强,说明原因?

（2）如果将颈动脉体麻醉后再吸入高浓度的 CO_2 和静脉注射乳酸,对呼吸运动的作用有何变化? 为什么?

（3）根据"观察项目"(6)(7)(8)中的实验结果,分析设计此实验的科研思路。

（寻庆英）

实验十六　尿生成的影响因素

【实验目的】

学习从膀胱引流尿液的方法,观察一些生理因素对尿生成量的影响。

【实验原理】

尿液的生成包括肾小球滤过、肾小管和集合管的重吸收以及分泌 3 个过程。其中,肾小球滤过的动力是肾小球有效滤过压,影响肾小球有效滤过压的因素包括肾小球毛细血管血压、血浆胶体渗透压和肾小囊内压,凡能影响这三者的因素都将影响肾脏的滤过功能。另外,肾小管溶液中的溶质的浓度以及抗利尿激素是影响肾小管和集合管重吸收的重要因素,这些因素的改变也会引起尿生成量的变化。

【实验材料】

（1）器材:RM6240 EC 多道生理信号采集处理系统、兔手术台、哺乳动物手术器械、气管插管、动脉插管、膀胱插管、血压换能器、记滴器、培养皿。

（2）药品:25%乌拉坦溶液、肝素(1 mg/kg)、25%葡萄糖溶液、1∶10 000 去甲肾上腺素溶液、呋塞米和垂体后叶素。

【实验对象】

家兔

【方法和步骤】

1. 手术操作

（1）抓兔和称重。

（2）沿耳缘静脉注射 25%乌拉坦(4 ml/kg)进行麻醉,以仰卧位固定于兔手术台上,保持静脉注射通路畅通。

（3）颈部剪毛,在颈前正中作一皮肤切口,分离皮下组织,钝性分离肌肉组织,暴露出气管并作气管插管以保持呼吸通畅。颈部手术暂时结束,用浸有生理盐水的纱布覆盖颈部创面,注意勿覆盖气管插管口。

（4）下腹部剪毛,于耻骨联合上方正中作一 3～5 cm 长切口,沿腹白线切开腹壁,将膀胱向尾侧移出体外,辨清楚膀胱的解剖位置,在顶端作一 1 cm 左右的切口,插入已注满水的膀胱插管,插管口尽量正对输尿管在膀胱的入口处,但不要紧贴膀胱后壁以防堵塞输尿管,用线沿切口结扎两道,将切口边缘固定在膀胱插管管壁凹陷处。手术结束后,用浸有生理盐水的纱布覆盖创面。

(5)分离颈部右侧迷走神经。

(6)分离出左侧颈总动脉,自耳缘静脉注射肝素溶液进行全身肝素化,再将肝素液充满动脉插管进行局部肝素化;然后进行颈总动脉插管。将动脉插管与血压换能器连接。手术结束后,用浸有生理盐水的纱布覆盖颈部创面,注意勿覆盖气管插管口。

2.实验装置的连接和使用

将血压换能器连接至 RM6240 EC 多道生理信号采集处理系统 3 通道接口,以正确描记血压。将从膀胱插管中流出的尿液滴在记滴器上,并将记滴器与系统通道 4 连接,用以记录尿的滴数。通过尿滴频率反应尿量的变化,将刺激电极与系统的刺激输出连接。

【观察项目】

(1)打开动脉夹以及膀胱插管弹簧夹,记录家兔正常血压及尿量。

(2)由家兔耳缘静脉快速注射生理盐水 20 ml,观察血压及尿量的变化。

(3)由家兔耳缘静脉快速注射 1∶10 000 去甲肾上腺素溶液 0.3 ml,观察血压及尿量的变化。

(4)经家兔耳缘静脉快速注射 25% 葡萄糖溶液 5 ml,观察血压及尿量的变化。

(5)电刺激迷走神经(刺激参数:刺激强度 5~10 V,刺激波宽 2 ms,刺激持续时间 5~10 s),观察血压和尿量变化。

(6)自耳缘静脉注射呋塞米(5 mg/kg),观察血压和尿量的变化。

(7)自耳缘静脉注射垂体后叶素(2U),观察血压和尿量的变化。

【注意事项】

(1)为保证动物在实验过程中有足够的尿液,实验前给动物喂食菜叶或手术过程中在动物腹腔注射 40 ml 生理盐水。

(2)手术尽量轻柔,腹部切口不可过大,以免体液损失较多影响尿量。

(3)实验过程中需多次静脉注射,所以应保护好兔耳缘静脉,注射进针时尽量从静脉远端开始。

(4)每项实验步骤须在上一项实验因素的作用消失后(即血压和尿量基本恢复至正常水平)再开始,以避免药物效应的相互干扰,并有益于了解药物作用的潜伏期、最大作用以及恢复期等信息。

(5)迷走神经刺激不宜过度,刺激时间不能太长,刺激强度不能太大,以免血压急剧下降,血压骤停。

【问题讨论】

"全身动脉血压升高,尿量一定增加,动脉血压降低,尿量一定减少"这句话对吗?为什么?

(杨健)

实验十七　呋塞米及高渗葡萄糖对尿液生成的影响

【实验目的】

观察呋塞米及高渗葡萄糖对水及电解质排泄的影响,了解利尿药及脱水药的实验方法。

【实验原理】

呋塞米作用于肾小管髓袢升支粗段皮质部和髓质部,抑制 $Na^+ - K^+ - 2Cl^-$ 共转运子,导致尿液中 Na^+、K^+、Cl^- 排出增多,肾的稀释功能减弱;并且由于髓质高渗压下降,降低了肾的浓缩功能,最终导致水的重吸收减少,排出大量尿液。呋塞米作用迅速、强大,持续时间短。脱水药静注后不易通过毛细血管进入组织,易经肾小球滤过,不被或少被肾小管重吸收,在肾小管几乎不代谢。常用的药物有 20% 的甘露醇,50% 的高渗葡萄糖溶液,而后者可部分从血管弥散进入组织中,并易被代谢,故作用弱不持久。

【实验材料】

(1) 器材:火焰光度计,手术台,手术器械一套,膀胱插管,导尿管,注射器(1 ml,10 ml,50 ml),蒸发皿,滴定管,烧杯,量筒。

(2) 药品:25%乌拉坦,50%葡萄糖溶液,1%呋塞米,$20\ \mu g/ml\ Na^+/K^+$ 标准溶液。

【实验对象】

家兔。

【实验步骤】

实验前按 50 ml/kg 给家兔温水灌胃,然后用 25%乌拉坦(4 ml/kg,1 g/kg)耳缘静脉注射麻醉,将家兔固定在兔台上手术。下腹部剪毛,由耻骨联合上缘沿正中线 3～5 cm 左右皮肤切口,再沿腹白线剪开腹壁及腹膜,暴露膀胱,沿膀胱壁避开血管作一个小切口,用注射器抽取膀胱中的尿液备用,再插入膀胱套管,套管口对准输尿管口,结扎固定。将膀胱和套管放回腹腔,用生理盐水纱布覆盖切口。

给药前每 5 min 收集尿液 1 次并记录尿量,共计 30 min。后续实验分两组,一组经耳缘静脉注射呋塞米 5 mg/kg;另一组经耳缘静脉注射 50%葡萄糖溶液 5 ml/kg。给完每种药物后,每 5 min 收集尿液并记录尿量,共计 30 min。

将给予生理盐水和不同药物后的尿液分别做如下处理以测定尿液中的 Na^+、K^+、Cl^- 的含量。

1. 用火焰光度计比较法测定尿液中 Na^+、K^+ 的含量

用 $20\ \mu g/ml\ Na^+/K^+$ 标准溶液校准火焰光度计。分别吸取给药前和给药后尿液各 0.2 ml,加入蒸馏水稀释至 30 ml(稀释倍数 150 倍),用火焰光度计分别测定稀释液中 Na^+ 和 K^+ 的浓度 A_x。尿液样本中 Na^+ 和 K^+ 的浓度 $C_x = A_x \times$ 稀释倍数(150);则 30 min 内的离子总量 = 离子浓度 $C_x \times$ 30 min 内的总尿量。

2. 用银滴定法测定尿液中 Cl^- 的含量

原理:用硝酸银试剂将尿液中的 Cl^- 沉淀为氯化银,所有的 Cl^- 都被沉淀完之后,若硝酸银一有过量,便与铬酸钾作用形成橘红色沉淀。

$$NaCl + AgNO_3 \rightarrow AgCl \downarrow + NaNO_3$$
$$2AgNO_3 + K_2CrO_4 \rightarrow Ag_2CrO_4 \downarrow + 2KNO_3$$

分别吸取给药前和给药后尿液各 1 ml,加蒸馏水稀释至 10 ml,加入 20% 铬酸钾溶液 2 滴,然后慢慢滴入硝酸银标准溶液(1 ml 相当于 0.606 mg 的 Cl^-),边滴边搅拌,至呈不褪色的橘红色为止。记录所消耗的硝酸银标准溶液体积(ml)。尿液中 Cl^- 的浓度:Cl^-(mg/ml)= 滴定时所消耗的硝酸银标准溶体积(ml)× 0.606 mg/ml ÷ 1 ml。则 30 min 内的 Cl^- 总量 = Cl^- 浓度 × 30 min 内的总尿量。实验结果分别填入表 3-14 和 3-15。

表 3-14 药物对家兔尿量的影响

药物	0~30 min 内尿量(ml)	每 5 min 内的尿量(ml)					
		0~5 (min)	5~10 (min)	10~15 (min)	15~20 (min)	20~25 (min)	25~30 (min)
用药前							
呋塞米 (或 50% 葡萄糖)							

表 3-15 药物对 Na^+、K^+、Cl^- 排泄的影响

药物	0~30 min 内尿量 (ml)	Na^+		K^+		Cl^-		
		浓度 (μg/ml)	总量 (mg)	浓度 (μg/ml)	总量 (mg)	硝酸银 (ml)	浓度 (mg/ml)	总量 (mg)
用药前								
呋塞米 (或 50% 葡萄糖)								

【注意事项】

(1)膀胱插管时避免结扎输尿管。

(2)若给药前未能收集到尿液,应以膀胱中原有尿液作为参比对照。

【问题讨论】

(1)利尿药和脱水药有哪些不同之处?

(2)绘制累积尿量随时间变化的折线图,并结合实验结果,分析尿液形成的机制。

(易宏伟)

实验十八　氨在肝性脑病发生机制中的作用

【实验目的】

通过急性肝功能不全动物模型的复制,探讨肝性脑病的发病机理及其治疗。

【实验原理】

(1)"肝蒂结扎"——肝脏原位去功能化。

(2)肠腔注入含 NH_4^+ 制剂,增高血氨(NH_3)浓度。

$$（水溶性）NH_4^+ \underset{[H^+]}{\overset{[OH^-]}{\Longleftrightarrow}} NH_3（脂溶性）$$

肠道吸收:难　　　　　　易

血脑屏障通透:难　　　　　易

3. 静脉注射谷氨酸钠制剂抢救。

$$谷氨酸 + NH_3 \Longleftrightarrow 谷氨酰胺$$

【实验材料】

(1)器材:兔台 1 个,腹部手术器械 1 套,5、20、50 ml 注射器各 1 只,导尿管 1 根。

(2)药品:1%利多卡因,2.5%氯化铵应用液(5%葡萄糖溶液 100 ml 中含 2.5 g 氯化铵和 1.5 g 碳酸氢钠),2.5%谷氨酸钠应用液(5%葡萄糖溶液 100 ml 中含 2.5 g 谷氨酸钠)。

【实验对象】

家兔。

【实验步骤】

1. 实验兔

(1)取家兔 1 只,称重后仰卧位固定在兔台上,剪去上腹部被毛,沿肋弓下缘 1 cm 处用利多卡因局部浸润麻醉。将充满生理盐水的头皮针刺入耳缘静脉备用。

(2)于剑突下 1 cm 处开始向两侧做与肋弓平行的弧形切口,长约 8 cm,打开腹腔,注意及时结扎较大的小血管,沿正中线两侧约 1 cm 处有腹壁上动、静脉上下走行,尤其需要注意及时结扎。

(3)打开腹腔后,将肝脏下压,暴露并小心剪断肝与横膈间镰状韧带;再将肝脏向上翻,分辨出肝胃韧带并小心将其剪断。

(4)找出十二指肠,在其上尽量避开血管做一直径近 1 cm 的小荷包缝合,在荷包缝合中央处用眼科剪剪一小口,将导尿管向空回肠方向插入约 3 cm,并收紧荷包,打结固定。

(5)以一粗线结扎肝左外叶、左中叶、右中叶和方形叶的根部,结扎时务必扎紧以确保上述几叶肝脏血流阻断,将肝肠等脏器纳入腹腔后以皮钳将腹壁创缘间夹紧,关腹。

（6）观察家兔的角膜反射,肌紧张程度以及对针刺疼痛的反应。

（7）由导管向十二指肠内缓缓注入氯化铵应用液,注意勿将此液漏入腹腔,首次剂量10 ml,2～3 min注完,以后每隔5 min缓慢注射5 ml,大约1 min注完,注意观察上述指标的变化,直至抽搐发生(注意区别动物挣扎与抽搐),记录此时所用氯化铵应用液的量,并计算出每千克体重用量,以便与对照兔进行比较。

（8）家兔刚出现抽搐,除立即停用氯化铵应用液外,需自耳缘静脉注入谷氨酸钠应用液（30 ml/kg）予以治疗,并记录治疗后上述指标的变化。

2．对照兔

除不做上述"步骤5"中肝结扎外,其余步骤均与实验兔相同,记录至抽搐出现时所用氯化铵应用液的量,算出每千克体重用量与实验兔比较,并观察下述各项指标。

角膜反射:用"＋"或"－"反映"存在"或"消失";

肌紧张程度:用"＋＋＋""＋＋"或"＋"反映"强""弱"程度;

疼痛反应:用"＋＋＋""＋＋""＋"或"－"反映"强""弱"程度;

抽搐:用"＋"或"－"反映"有"或"无"。

表 3-16 　氨在肝性脑病发生机制中作用的实验观察

氯化铵用量（ml）	对照兔				实验兔			
	角膜反射	肌紧张程度	疼痛反应	抽搐	角膜反射	肌紧张程度	疼痛反应	抽搐
10								
15								
20								
25								
30								
35								
40								
45								
50								
55								
60								
治疗后								
每千克体重 NH_4Cl 用量								

【注意事项】

（1）动物先称重。固定动物一定要固定牢。

（2）动物仅采用局部麻醉,以手术时动物不挣扎为准。开腹后动作轻柔,不要将肝戳破以致失血性休克。

（3）在上腹部手术时，应注意防止大量出血。

（4）小荷包缝合后将缝针夹于持针器上。

（5）注意保持药物抢救通路（耳缘静脉）通畅。

（6）插入导尿管方向为空回肠方向，请勿反方向插入。

【问题讨论】

（1）本实验中，为什么实验兔结扎肝蒂后，经十二指肠注入碱性氯化氨溶液可诱发家兔"脑病"？

（2）本实验中，为什么对照兔未结扎肝蒂，经十二指肠注入碱性氯化氨溶液也可诱发家兔"脑病"？

（3）为什么应用谷氨酸钠可治疗肝性脑病？

（廖凯　沈传陆）

实验十九　心血管活动的神经体液调节

【实验目的】

（1）学习哺乳动物动脉血压的直接测量和记录方法。

（2）通过观察动脉血压，分析神经-体液因素对心血管活动的调节。

【实验原理】

在生理情况下，哺乳动物动脉血压相对稳定，这种相对稳定是通过神经、体液因素的调节实现。神经调节中以颈动脉窦-主动脉弓压力感受器反射（降压反射）尤为重要。

（1）血压的神经调节（降压反射）：降压反射调节可在血压升高时发挥降压作用，在血压降低时发挥升压作用。此反射的传入神经为主动脉神经和窦神经。家兔的主动脉神经为独立的一条神经，称降压神经。

（2）血压的体液调节：

心血管活动还受肾上腺素和去甲肾上腺素等体液因素的调节。肾上腺素对 α 与 β_1 及 β_2 受体均有激活作用，引起心输出量增加。去甲肾上腺素主要激活 α 受体而对 β_2 受体作用很小，因而使外周阻力增加，动脉血压升高，但对心脏的作用要比肾上腺素弱。乙酰胆碱可与 M 受体结合引起心输出量的减少。

本实验通过血压换能器把压力转化为电信号，输入到计算机。

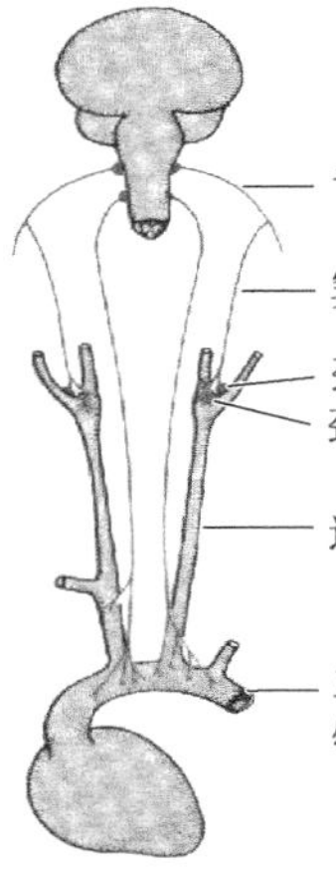

——舌咽神经

——窦神经

——颈动脉体
颈动脉窦

——迷走神经

——主动脉弓压力感受器

图 3-10　颈动脉窦-主动脉弓压力感受器系统

【实验材料】

（1）器材：RM6240 EC 多道生理信号采集处理系统，哺乳动物手术器械 1 套，兔手术操作台，血压换能器，气管插管，玻璃分针,注射器(20ml,2ml),动脉插管,动脉夹,头皮针,棉线,细丝线。

（2）药品:生理盐水,25%乌拉坦,1%肝素,1:10 000 肾上腺素,1:10 000 去甲肾上腺素,1:10 000 乙酰胆碱。

【实验对象】

家兔。

【实验步骤】

1. 家兔称重、麻醉与固定

用25%乌拉坦(4 ml/kg,1 g/kg)从家兔耳缘静脉缓慢注入,动物麻醉的标志为四肢松软、疼痛反射消失、角膜反射消失、呼吸变深变慢。麻醉后用绳子将动物背位固定于兔手术台上。

2. 颈部手术

（1）气管插管:剪去颈部兔毛(从甲状软骨到胸骨上缘间),在颈部沿正中线切开皮肤约5～7 cm,用止血钳分离皮下组织和肌肉,暴露气管。游离气管,在距甲状软骨2～3 cm处切开气管(倒"T"形切口),往肺脏方向插入气管插管并固定。

（2）分离右侧颈动脉鞘内容物:仔细区分颈总动脉鞘内的3根神经,其中迷走神经最粗,减压神经最细,颈交感神经居中。用玻璃分针将神经按由细到粗的顺序依次分离,并用不同颜色的丝线进行标记。最后分离颈总动脉并用棉线标记。血管和神经的分离应操作轻柔,而且分离顺序应先神经后血管、由细到粗。

（3）动脉插管:将左侧颈总动脉游离2 cm,按照体重1 ml/kg的剂量从家兔耳缘静脉注射浓度1%的肝素进行全身血液抗凝。然后,颈总动脉远心端用棉线结扎,近心端用动脉夹夹闭。用眼科剪在颈总动脉上靠近结扎线处剪一切口,往心脏方向插入充满肝素的动脉插管,再用棉线将其固定至颈总动脉(切勿打开近心端动脉夹)。

3. 实验装置连接

将动脉插管连接血压换能器。将血压换能器固定在万能支台上,其输出端连接到计算机通道上。打开近心端动脉夹。

【观察项目】

（1）描记正常的动脉血压曲线,观察一级波、二级波。动脉血压随心室的收缩和舒张而变化:心室收缩时血压上升,心室舒张时血压下降,这种血压随心动周期波动称为心搏波(一级波),其频率与心率一致;同时,动脉血压也随呼吸运动而变化,吸气时血压先下降后上升,呼气时先上升后下降,这种波叫呼吸波(二级波),其频率与呼吸节律一致。

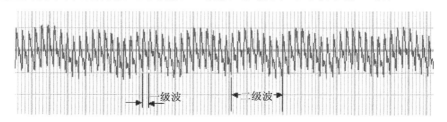

图 3-11　正常动脉血压波形

（2）用动脉夹夹闭右侧颈总动脉 10～15 s,观察动脉血压有何变化。

（3）用保护电极刺激右侧完整的降压神经（刺激强度 3～5 V,频率 10～20 Hz,刺激波宽 5 ms,刺激持续时间 5～10 s),观察动脉血压有何变化。

（4）用保护电极刺激右侧迷走神经外周端（刺激参数同上）,观察动脉血压有何变化。

（5）从耳缘静脉注入 1:10 000 的肾上腺素 0.3 ml,观察动脉血压有何变化。

（6）从耳缘静脉注入 1:10 000 去甲肾上腺素 0.3 ml,观察动脉血压有何变化。

（7）从耳缘注入 1:10 000 的乙酰胆碱 0.3 ml,观察动脉血压有何变化。

【注意事项】

（1）麻醉过程要熟练掌握,避免麻醉过量。

（2）整个实验过程中,均需保持动脉插管与动脉平行,以免刺破动脉。

（3）每项观察都待血压恢复正常,才能进行下一个项目观察。

（4）每次注射药物之后,立即用一注射器静脉注入 0.5 ml 生理盐水,以防药液残留在针头及局部静脉中影响下一种药物作用。

【问题讨论】

（1）短时夹闭对侧颈总动脉对全身血压有何影响？为什么？假如夹闭部位在颈动脉窦以上,影响是否相同？

（2）刺激迷走神经,对动脉血压有何影响？为什么？

（成于思）

实验二十　药物对麻醉家兔急性心衰血流动力学的影响

【实验目的】

（1）掌握实时测量血流动力学指标和致急性心衰模型的方法。

（2）观察药物对麻醉家兔血流动力学的影响。

【实验原理】

心力衰竭是指在适度的静脉回心血量下,心排出量的绝对或相对减少,不能满足机体组织需要的一种病理状态。

心力衰竭的临床症状包括由于心输出量不足引起的乏力、运动能力下降、心动过速、劳力性呼吸困难、紫绀、低血压等,以及由于回心血量减少引起静脉高压,其症状主要表现为下肢肿胀、腹水、肝脾肿大、颈静脉怒张、肺水肿(肺部罗音)、端坐呼吸、呼吸困难等。

临床诊断心力衰竭除了根据临床症状和体征外,还可以根据左心射血指数(LVEF),当 LVEF≤40%～50%,可诊断为左室收缩功能不全。近年来,有人认为 BNP(B 型利钠肽)>400 ng/L 或 NT-proBNP(N 末端 B 型利钠肽原)>1 500 ng/L,可诊断心衰(阳性率 90%)。治疗后 BNP/NT-proBNP 显著降低≥30%～50%,提示治疗有效。

血流动力学参数：

（1）心率（HR）。

（2）动脉血压（BP）：收缩压（SBP），舒张压（DBP）和平均动脉压（MAP）。

（3）心肌收缩性能指标：

① 左室收缩压（LVSP）；

② 左室压最大上升速度（dp/dt max）：dp/dt 为测取心室内压变化的速率指标，在一定程度上可间接反映心室收缩时室壁张力变化的大小，其峰值 +dp/dt max 代表心室等容收缩期结束时瞬间室内压升高的最大速率，在主动脉瓣开放前瞬间到达，它是评定心肌收缩性能的常用指标，对收缩性能急速改变敏感，但受负荷影响较大；

③ $t-dp/dt$ max：左心室开始收缩至最大收缩速率时间，一般时间越短，心脏收缩功能越好。

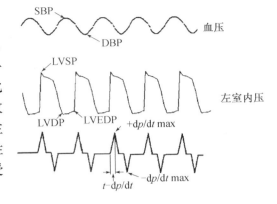

图 3-12　血压与心室内压波形示意图

（4）心肌舒张性能指标

① 左室压最大下降速度（-dp/dt max）：-dp/dt max 代表心室等容舒张期结束时瞬间室内压下降的最大速率，在二尖瓣开放前瞬间到达；

② 等容舒张期左室压下降的时间常数（T 值）；

③ 左室舒张压（LVDP）；

④ 左室舒张末期压（LVEDP）。

【实验材料】

（1）器材：手术器械 1 套，家兔手术台，RM6240 EC 多道生理信号采集处理系统，聚乙烯塑料心导管和动脉插管，注射器，烧杯，天平。

（2）药品：生理盐水，25% 乌拉坦，1% 和 0.1% 肝素，0.1% 维拉帕米，0.01% 去甲肾上腺素，0.002 5% 西地兰（毛花苷 C），0.5% 氨茶碱，0.002% 多巴酚丁胺，1% 呋塞米等。

【实验对象】

家兔，体重 1.8～2.5 kg，雌雄不拘。

【实验步骤】

（1）打开信号处理器和电脑电源，点击电脑屏幕上的 RM6240 EC 多道生理信号采集处理系统。

（2）从"实验（X）"中选择"血流动力学"。

（3）点击右上方菜单"开始观察（▶）"。

（4）检查血压管道信号是否畅通：用手捏压充满水的橡胶管，观察屏幕上相应通道的扫描线是否有相应反应。

（5）取1只家兔，称重。耳缘静脉注射25%乌拉坦麻醉（4 ml/kg，1 g/kg），麻醉后仰卧固定于手术台上。

正中切开颈部皮肤，分离两侧颈总动脉。穿线、结扎远心端，留一线在近心端以备结扎固定。用动脉夹夹住近心端，用眼科剪在颈动脉上剪一小口，并插入含有0.1%肝素的聚乙烯导管，从家兔右颈总动脉把心导管插入心室（以血压波变成心室内压波为进入心室的指标），描记心室内压。

从家兔左颈总动脉把动脉导管插入，描记血压。两插管用线扎紧固定。"通道1"选择血压测量。"通道2"选择心室内压，"通道3"为心室内压的微分波。在相应通道中选择动态实时测量，观察各参数的正常值。手术完毕后稳定10 min。

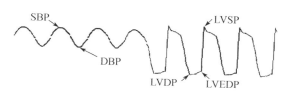

图3-13　心导管从颈动脉插入心室时的压力波形变化

（6）实验正式开始：选择并点击"记录"。

（7）标记：输入需要标记的文字或符号，如"去甲肾上腺素"，在注射药物去甲肾上腺素时点击标记。观察注射药物后变化的起始位置。

（8）家兔急性心衰模型的建立：

方法一：给家兔耳缘静脉快速注射大量生理盐水5～8 ml/kg·min，注射5 min。注射后观察10 min，以家兔出现呼吸急促，左室压最大上升速度（dp/dt max）下降40%～50%为心衰指标。

如没有出现心衰，可选择方法二。

方法二：静脉注射去甲肾上腺素（0.01%）1.0 ml/kg，观察10 min，观察急性心衰的症状和体征。

如果仍然没有出现心衰，可选择方法三。

方法三：缓慢注射0.1%维拉帕米0.2 ml/kg，边注射边观察急性心衰的症状和体征。

（9）出现心衰后，分别给予西地兰、氨茶碱、多巴酚丁胺、呋塞米等药物进行抢救，给药量均为1.0 ml/kg。每注射一种药物后观察10 min，比较这些药物对各项参数的影响，解释它们的作用机制。

（10）实验完毕后，要给本次实验文件起名，存盘。

（11）实验数据的阅读和选择：

在相应的文件中阅读和截取实验数据。用实验分析栏中的"标记查寻"，或压缩实验图形，找到你所需要的实验数据段。选择相应通道的静态测量，压力（"通道1"选择血压测量，"通道2"选择心室内压测量）选择平均值、手动测量和相应的参数。计算机可以自动给出相应时段的实验数据。然后可以导出Word文件或Excel文件，裁剪编辑实验结果，用于实验报告。

实验结果填入表3-17。

表 3-17　实验结果

药　物	SP	DP	HR	LVSP	LVDP	$+\mathrm{d}p/\mathrm{d}t$ max	$-\mathrm{d}p/\mathrm{d}t$ max	$t-\mathrm{d}p/\mathrm{d}t$ max
正常								
生理盐水								
去甲肾上腺素								
维拉帕米								
多巴酚丁胺								
西地兰								
氨茶碱								
呋塞米								

【注意事项】

（1）插管时动作要轻、慢，以免刺破血管，同时观察计算机显示屏上血压波的变化，来判断是否插入心室。

（2）如血压波消失成一直线，心导管不能继续向前插，须后退直到压力波出现后可改变转动方向继续前插。管子如有折断应该更换。

（3）实验完毕后要及时存盘（标记自己班级和时间），读取相应数据作为实验结果，进行实验分析。

【问题讨论】

（1）造成心衰的实验方法有哪几种？解释其原理。

（2）西地兰、多巴酚丁胺、氨茶碱、呋塞米等治疗急性心衰的机制是什么？

（3）评价心脏收缩功能的指标有哪几个？它们的含义是什么？

（吴晓冬）

Experiment 1　Basic surgery procedures on experimental animals

Experimental purpose

（1）To understand the importance and ABC features of functional experiments.

（2）To understand the laboratory regulations and requirements.

（3）To master the targeted requirements for operating functional experiment,

（4）To study how to write the lab report.

Experimental materials

（1）Instruments:metal instruments; non-metal instruments in Table 3-1.

Table 3-1　Instruments in the experiment

Metal Instruments (in Metal plate)		Non-metla instrumentscin Plastic plote	
Item	Quantity	Item	Quantity
Scissors (curved, straight)	2	Scalp acupuncture	1
Forceps	4	Glass dissecting needle	2
Hemostatic forceps	3	Thick rope	4
Bulldog-clamp	2	Silk thread	3
Eye scissors	1	Cotton thread	1
Eye tweezers	1	Fine rope	1
Pinhead	1	Feather	1
Non-metal instruments (in Plastic plate)		Trachea cannula	1
		Arterial cannula	1
Item	Quantity	Bladder cannula	1
Porcelain-cup	1	Plastic cup	1
Gauze	4	Syringes (20 ml; 2 ml)	2

（2）Drugs:25% urethane, 1% heparin.

Experimental subjects

Rabbit

Experimental procedures

1. Pre-surgery Preparations

（1）Holding a rabbit: One hand grips the scruff of the neck firmly,the other hand holds the buttock of the rabbit.

（2）Weighing: put the rabbit on the platform balance to measure the body weight. If the rabbit is not quiet and moves around, we can calm it down by gently touching its back skin. In this way, we can get the body weight easily.

（3）Anesthesia: 25% urethane is given slowly to rabbits at the dose of 4 ml/kg through the pinna marginal vein. The depth of anesthesia should be monitored by observing the following 4 signs:

Pain reflex- pinching the toe or foot web with hemostasis will cause a pain response. Limb withdraws in response to pinching is a sign that the anesthesia is not deep enough. If withdraw is not seen, it indicates that the animal cannot sense the pain.

Corneal reflex- Corneal reflex can be induced by touching the cornea of the eye with a piece of soft feather. This touch should result in blinking when the animal is awake (corneal reflex). Once the animal shows no corneal reflex, it is likely that the animal has been anesthetized deep enough for operation.

Muscle tone- Test muscle tone by pulling the limbs of the animal. Rigid muscle indicates inadequate depth of anesthesia. If the muscles are fully relaxed, the depth of anesthesia is adequate.

Monitor cardiopulmonary function and body temperature- If an animal is anesthetized too deeply, its respiration rate and cardiac output will decrease, resulting in low blood oxygenation, low blood pressure, poor tissue perfusion and low body temperature.

(4) Restraining: Rabbits should be restrained with cotton ropes in supine position on the operation table.

2. Operation procedures

1) Operation in neck region

(1) Shearing: Shear off the hair in the anterior region of the neck with one pair of curved scissors.

(2) Skin incision: Make a middle line skin incision of $5\sim7$ cm using a pair of straight scissors on ventral neck starting to expose the underneath structures by pulling skin aside using 4 forceps along the diagonal direction.

(3) Separating the subcutaneous tissue: Make an incision in the subcutaneous tissue like that in the skin.

(4) Blunt separating the muscles with two pairs of hemostasis alternatively in order to expose the trachea.

(5) Trachea intubation: Isolate and free trachea from surrounding soft tissue and make an inverted "T" shape incision on the trachea $2\sim3$ cm under the throat. Insert the tracheal cannula toward the lung and tie the cannula to the trachea.

(6) Isolating the right depressor nerve, vagus nerve and common carotid artery.

Carefully identify the three nerves that are located in carotid sheath: vagus nerve is the thickest, depressor nerve is the thinnest and the sympathetic nerve is in between in its diameter. Isolate them by opening the sheath bluntly using a glass dissecting needle. Put threads of different colors under each of them for easy identification. Finally, dissect the common carotid artery and mark it with a piece of cotton thread. The actions of isolating blood vessels and nerves should be gentle. It is recommended to isolate the thinnest depressor nerve first.

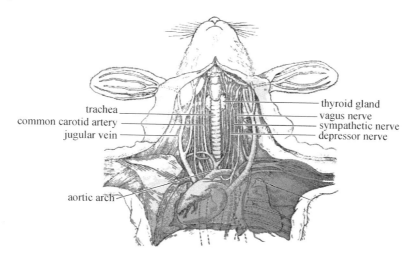

Figure 3-1 Dissociation of xiphoid process

（7）Intubation of the left common carotid artery: Isolate and free the left carotid artery by 2 cm. Inject the rabbit with 1% heparin via earmarginal vein at a dose of 1 ml/kg to anti-coagulate the blood. Then, tie a knot in the distal end of the isolated segment with a piece of cotton thread and clip the other end with a bulldog clamp. Make a small incision close to the aforementioned knot in the isolated artery with a pair of eye scissors. Insert an arterial cannula filled with 1% heparin into the artery in the direction toward the heart and tie it up with the artery.

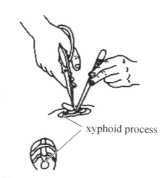

Figure 3-2 Cervical and pectoral anatomy of the rabbit

2) Operation in upper belly

Make an incision of 2 cm through the skin and subcutaneous tissue along the middle line of the upper belly. Cut open the muscle of the *abdominal wall along linea alba abdominis and* the peritoneum to expose the xiphoid process. Cut off the sternum body, and then hook up the xiphoid process with a pin hook connected with a piece of thread.

3) Operation in the lower belly

Make an incision through the skin and subcutaneous tissue along the middle line above the symphysis pubis. Cut open the muscle of *abdominal wall along linea alba abdominis and* the abdominal cavity to expose the bladder. Make a cut of 0.5 cm in diameter at the summit of the bladder and insert the bladder cannula filled with water into the bladder. Tie the cannula with a piece of cotton thread to the bladder at the entrance.

Notices

(1) Urethane is given through the pinna marginal vein slowly; fast administration can inhibit the respiration of the rabbit and induce death.

(2) The actions of separating blood vessels and nerves should be gentle. Avoid using metal instruments when separating nerves.

Questions and discussion

(1) Based on the protocol of operation on the rabbit, how can you intubate the ureter to record the urine formation?

(2) Why should the surgical operation bestandardized ?

(Xiaoniu Dai)

Experiment 2   Effects of different dosage on drug action

Experimental purpose

(1) To learn the method of restraint and handling the mice and the procedures of intraperitoneal injection.

(2) To observe the effects of different doses of amobarbital sodium on mice.

Experimental principles

Amobarbital sodium has an extensive inhibitory effect on central nervous system. Administration of high dosage of amobarbital sodium will cause sedation, lypnosis, anticonvulsion and narcotism symptoms in experimental animals, while the medium dosage may cause hypnosis. To determine the effect of amobarbital sodium on hypnosis, we will examine the righting reflex of animals, which will adjust the orientation of the body when it is taken out of its normal upright position. Once the righting reflex disappears, it means the animals are induced to hypnosis by amobarbital sodium.

Experimental materials

(1) Instruments: bell jar, balance, syringes(1 ml).

(2) Drugs: 0.3% and 0.9% amobarbital sodium

Experimental subjects

Two mice (Kun Ming), weighing about 18~22 g.

Experimental procedures

(1) Hold and weigh 2 mice. One is injected intraperitoneally with 0.3% amobarbital sodium (30 mg/kg), and the other is injected intraperitoneally with 0.9% amobarbital sodium (90 mg/kg). Observe the activities of the mice after injecting, record the time point when the mice start to lose righting reflex and calculate the latency to onset of action as well as the duration of action.

(2) Observation items: righting reflex disappear. (If the mice could maintain arms and legs up more than one minute, the response of righting reflex disappear is positive,

otherwise it is negative.)

(3) Fill the experimental results in table 3-2.

Table 3-2　Effects of different doses of amobarbital sodium on mice

Mouse number	Weight (g)	Dose (mg/kg)	Onset time of righting reflex disappear(min)	Duration of righting reflex disappear (min)
1				
2				

Notices

(1) Insert the syringe needle subcutaneously first and then into the abdominal cavity in a 45 degree angle when performing intraperitoneal injection.

(2) In order to avoid getting into thoracic cavity, please do not make your injection position too high.

Questions and discussion

What are the effects of different doses of amobarbital sodium on the righting reflex in mice? Explain this result.

(*Lei Zhao*)

Experiment 3　Effects of different administration routes on drug action

1. Effects of different administration routes of amobarbital sodium on mice

Experimental purpose

To observe the effects of different administration routes of amobarbital sodium on mice.

Experimental principles

Drug absorption is affected by different administration routes, therefore influencing the onset and effectiveness of a drug.

Experimental materials

(1) Instruments: bell jar, balance, syringes(1 ml).

(2) Drugs: 1% amobarbital sodium.

Experimental subjects

Four mice (Kun Ming), weighing about 18~22 g.

Experimental procedures

Hold and weigh 4 mice. Divide them into 2 groups, each group has 2 mice. The first group of mice is injected intraperitoneally with 1% amobarbital sodium (100 mg/kg), and the other group is administrated intragastrically with 1% amobarbital sodium (100 mg/kg). Observe the activities of the mice after administration and record the time point when the righting reflex of the mice start to disappear and calculate the latency of action as well as the duration of action.

Observation items: righting reflex disappear. Fill the experimental results in table 3-3.

Table 3-3　Effects of different administration routes of amobarbital sodium on mice

Mouse number	Weight (g)	Administration route	Onset time of righting reflex disappear(min)	Duration of righting reflex disappear(min)
1				
2				
3				
4				

Notices

In intragastrical administration in a mouse, the mouse will be hold with oesophagus as straight as possible. Inset the needle carefully along the bent tube between the mouth and the oesophagus. Ensure that the drug is administered to the stomach smoothly. Wrong injections(e.g. into the lungs) usually cause immediate death.

Questions and discussion

What are the effects of different administration routes of amobarbital sodium on the righting reflex in mice? Explain this result.

2. Effects of different administration routes of magnesium sulfate on rabbits

Experimental purpose

Observe the effects of different administration routes of magnesium sulfate on rabbits.

Experimental principles

Magnesium sulfate is a common pharmaceutical preparation of magnesium administrated orally and intravenously. Oral magnesium sulfate is commonly used as a saline laxative or osmotic purgative, because it is difficult to absorb in the intestinal tract and causes a high osmotic environment to inhibit the water absorption leading to the increase volume of the intestinal tract and stimulate the peristalsis. However, while used intravenously, magnesium ion could specifically compete with calcium ion and inhibit its effect which therefore causes skeletal muscle, myocardium and vascular smooth muscle flaccidity, and because of that, magnesium sulfate has the effect of relaxing muscle flaccidity and lowering blood pressure.

Experimental materials

(1) Instruments: rabbit box, infant scale, syringes(5、10、50 ml).

(2) Drugs: 5% magnesium sulfate, 2.5% calcium chloride.

Experimental subjects

New Zealand, Two rabbits, weighing about 2.5kg.

Experimental procedures

Restrain and weigh two rabbits. One is injected intravenously with 5% magnesium sulfate (175 mg/kg) in the marginal vein, and the other is administrated intragastrically with the same dose of magnesium sulfate. Then observe the breathing, muscle tension, and feces of the rabbits. If the rabbit appears anhelation or muscle tension is down, inject intravenously with 2.5% calcium chloride (50 mg/kg) immediately. Fill the experimental results in Table 3-4.

Table 3-4　Effects of different administration routes of magnesium sulfate on rabbits

Rabbit number	Weight (kg)	Administration route of magnesium sulfate	Dose (mg/kg)	Breathing	Muscle tension	Feces
1						
2						

Notices

Range of safety of magnesium sulfate is very narrow, overdose will inhibit respiration, suddenly decrease blood pressure, and cause death. Inject slowly during intravenous injection.

Questions and discussion

What different responses will the rabbits have if they are treated with magnesium sulfate through different administration routes? Why?

(*Lei Zhao*)

Experiment 4　Determination of ED_{50}

Experimental purpose

(1) To observe the effects of different doses of sodium pentobarbital on mice.

(2) To learn the method of ED_{50} calculation.

Experimental principles

The magnitude of the drug effect depends on its dose. The potency of a drug is most easily analyzed by plotting the magnitude of the response versus the logarithm of the drug dose, thus obtaining a graded dose-response curve. The curve shows shape of "S" if the percentage response as Y axon and logarithms of dose as X axon, The slope where the response is 50% is greatest, and the most sensible point in dose-response curve. So we call logarithms of the dose as median effective dose, ED_{50}.

It is necessary to search for appropreciate range of dose before exact measurement of ED_{50}. It is also said that the dose which percentage response of mice approaches 0%

or 100% must be preliminarily tested. Then choose suitable ratio $(1:0.8\sim1:0.7)$ of dose in order to further determine the doses of various groups measured ED_{50}.

Experimental materials

(1) Instruments: bell jar, balance, syringes (1 ml).

(2) Drugs: sodium pentobarbital $(0.245\%, 0.196\%, 0.156\%, 0.125\%, 0.1\%)$

Experimental subjects

50 mice (Kun Ming), weighing about $18\sim22$ g.

Experimental procedures

(1) Divide the 50 mice into 5 groups, and 10 mice per group. Every group is injected intraperitoneally with different doses of the sodium pentobarbital. The doses are 49, 39, 31, 25 and 20 mg/kg respectively.

(2) Observation items: righting reflex disappear. (If the mice could maintain arms and legs up more than one minute, the response of righting reflex disappear is positive, otherwise it is negative.)

Fill the experimental results in table 3-5.

Table 3-5 Determiuation of ED50

Group	Dosage (mg/kg)	Total mice	Hypnotic mice	ED_{50} (mg/kg)
1	49	10		
2	39	10		
3	31	10		
4	25	10		
5	20	10		

(3) Calculating ED_{50}:

$$ED_{50} = \log^{-1}[X_m - I(\sum P - 0.5)]$$

X_m represents the logarithms of the Maximum dose

I represents ratio between doses

$\sum P$ represents the sum of each positive rate

Notices

Weigh and administer accurately, arrange mice group randomly

Questions and discussion

What is the clinical significance of determining ED_{50}, LD_{50} and TI of a drug?

(*Lei Zhao*)

Experiment 5 Identification of blood type in ABO group

Experimental purpose

To learn the methods and working principles of ABO blood type identification.

Experimental principles

The blood types of erythrocytes are determined by specific antigens of the cells. The ABO system is the most important blood-group system in human-blood transfusion. To ensure the safety of patients, blood types in ABO group must be identified before blood transfusion. The ABO blood types are made up of antigens located on the surface of erythrocyte and antibodies in the serum. In terms of blood type antibodies, type A individuals always have anti-B antibodies in their blood plasma. Similarly, type B individuals have anti-A antibodies, type AB individuals have neither anti-A nor anti-B antibody, and type O individuals have both anti-A and anti-B antibodies. Hemagglutination reaction will occur when an antigen encounters with its corresponding antibody. Therefore, the ABO type of an unknown blood sample can be determined by observing hemagglutination reaction using known standard serum antibodies as shown in Table 3-6.

Table 3-6 Antigens and antibodies in ABO blood group

Blood type	Antigens on red blood cells	Antibodies in serum
O	none	A and B
A	A antigen only	B only
B	B antigen only	A only
AB	A and B antigen	none

Experimental materials

Blood taking needle, glass slide with two wells, medical cotton (sterilized), small bamboo sticks (toothpick), dish, tray, microscope, 75% alcohol cotton, standard serum A and B.

Experimental subjects

Human Volunteer.

Experimental procedures

(1) Take a clean and dry glass slide. There are two ring-shape wells (umbilications) on the slide. Label it with A and B respectively.

(2) Drop one drop of anti-A or anti-B standard serum in each well labeled A and B respectively.

(3) Swab the skin site for taking blood (usually the earlobe of others or the left hand ring finger of yourself) with 75% alcohol cotton, wait until the alcohol evaporates. Pinch the skin with blood taking needle. Dispose the needle into the dirt bucket.

(4) Squeeze the finger or earlobe to get blood. Move one drop of blood into one well with the bamboo stick. Mix the blood with the antibody plasm in the well gently with the stick. Note, use one end of the stick for the blood in one well and avoid crossover of antibodies.

(5) Stop the bleeding by pressing a ball of dry cotton on the site of pinching.

(6) At room temperature, wait for $1\sim2$ minutes and observe with the naked eye whether the blood aggregates. If aggregation occurs only in well A or B, it is a type A or B blood. If aggregation is seen in both wells, it is an AB type blood. If no aggregation on either well it is a type O blood.

(7) Clean the used slides. Discard the used alcohol cotton balls, blood taking needles, toothpicks.

Notices

(1) Use only strictly sterilized needle for blood taking. Do not reuse any needles, especially, do not use a needle that has been used on another person.

(2) Make sure that the standard serums must not be confused. The separated end of the toothpick must be clearly dedicated for moving the blood to and mixing in the separated well.

(3) Inadequate blood may result in an ambitious result.

Questions and discussion

(1) According to your blood type, do you know which blood type(s) you can accept for blood transfusion and individuals with which blood type (s) can accept your blood? Why?

(2) If the standard A and B serums are not available, can you determine one's blood type by using another person's blood with known blood type (A or B)?

(*Lijuan Shi*)

Experiment 6　Auscultation of heart sounds

Experimental purpose

(1) To learn the method of auscultation of heart sounds.

(2) To know the characteristics of normal heart sounds.

Experimental principles

The cardiovascular system of a human being consists of the heart and blood vessels that are arranged to form double circulations: the systemic circulation and the pulmonary circulation. The normal blood flow through the heart and blood vessels is unidirectional. The flow of blood is driven by the pumping of the heart muscle and the unidirectional feature is established by four one-way valves. When the heart beats, the valves open and close to guide the blood flow in correct direction. The opening and closing of the four cardiac valves and the resulting turbulence of the blood flow produce sounds that can be heard on the body surface. In cardiac auscultation, an examiner uses a stethoscope to listen the sounds in order to obtain important information about the condition of the heart. Figure 3-3 depicts areas on the chest at which sounds produced by different parts of heart are heard best with the aid of stethoscope.

In healthy adults, there are mainly two normal heart sounds that occur in sequence

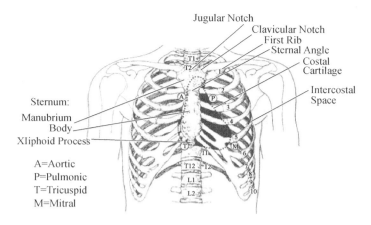

Figure 3-3   Auscultatory areas

with each heart beat. The first heart sound (S1) is caused by the sudden blockage of the reversed blood flow from ventricles to atria due to closure of the atrioventricular valves (mitral and tricuspid) at the beginning of ventricular contraction. When the pressure in the ventricles rises above the pressure in the atria, the blood flow entering the ventricles is pushed back toward the atria. Closing of the atrioventricular valves prevents the regurgitation of blood from the ventricles back into the atria. The closure causes the turbulence of the blood and the vibration of the valve to produce S1. The second heart sound (S2) is caused by the sudden blockage of the aortic valve and pulmonary valve at the end of ventricular systole. This blockage of the valves prevents the reversing of the blood flow from backing to the ventricles during ventricular diastole. The S2 is resulted from the blood turbulence caused by the sudden blockage of blood flow reversal. The characteristic first and second heart sounds produced by the heart are usually referred to as the 'lub-dup' sounds. The lower-pitched 'lub' is for S1 and the higher-pitched 'dup' is for S2.

Experimental materials

Stethoscopes.

Experimental subjects

Human volunteer.

Experimental procedures

(1) The volunteer sits quietly for 10 minutes before testing.

(2) The tester should pay attention to the direction of the earpiece insertion which must be consistent with the direction of the external ear canal when wearing stethoscope.

(3) The tester should adjust the position of the bell of the stethoscope to find the best position for clearest heart sound detection and to identify the two heart sounds carefully.

(4) Record your observation.

79

Heart rate

Observation items: Identify the two heart sounds carefully.

Notices

(1) The sounds are soft and therefore room noise must be kept to minimum.

(2) The earpiece must be insert forward to be in consistent with the direction of ear canal which runs slightly anteriorally. To avoid the spirant influence that generate by pipe friction, one should avoid the crossing of the two connecting pipes.

(3) If you cannot clearly hear the sounds, you can ask the testee to stop breathing for a moment when you listen.

Questions and discussion

How is the first heart sound and second heart sounds formed? What is the clinical significance of the two sounds?

(*Lijuan Shi*)

Experiment 7　Arterial blood pressure measurements

Experimental purpose

(1) To study the indirect measure of arterial blood pressure.

(2) To know the normal value of arterial blood pressure.

Experimental principles

The blood pressure (BP) in the arteries varies during the cardiac cycle. The ventricles contract to push blood into the arterial system, causing a sudden increase in BP, which slowly declines until the heart contracts again. BP is at its highest value immediately after the ventricle contracts (systolic pressure) and at its lowest value immediately prior to the ventrile contracts or the end of the ventricle diastole (diastolic pressure). Systolic and diastolic pressures can be measured by inserting a small catheter into an artery and connecting the catheter to a pressure gauge so that the BP can be measured by a pressure sensor. Such a direct measurement provides accurate values for BP, but the method is invasive, which limits its use in clinic. Noninvasive methods (usually indirect) with acceptable accuracy is recommended for clinical use.

Traditionally, arterial BP is estimated by an indirect method using a stethoscope and a blood pressure cuff that is connected to a mercury column or other sphygmomanometer. Examiners estimate the BP by listening to the sound quality changes with the blood flow change when the cuff pressure reduces. No sound can be heard when the blood flows through intravascular without any obstacle. In this case, the blood is in a pattern of laminar flow. But if a pressure is applied (via the cuff) outside the blood vessel, turbulence flow may occur which causes sound to be produced when the blood flow pass through the narrow part of the vessel. During the indirect measurement, the examiner fills the cuff to a pressure well above the systolic pressure of the testee and then releases the air slowly to drop off the pressure. When the pressure is just below the diastolic pressure, the blood starts to flow through interruptedly and sound can be heard. With the pressure further dropping off towards the diastole pressure, the quality of the sound will be changed.

Experimental materials

stethoscopes, sphygmomanometer.

Experimental subjects

Human volunteer.

Experimental procedures

(1) The volunteer sits quietly and relaxes for 5 minutes.

(2) The volunteer undresses the right (or left) sleeve and puts the arm on the table slightly making sure that the center of the upper arm is at the same height with the heart.

(3) Place the blood pressure cuff around the upper portion of the arm of the volunteer, between the elbow and the shoulder.

(4) Place the bell of the stethoscope over the brachial artery, as shown in following Figure 3-4.

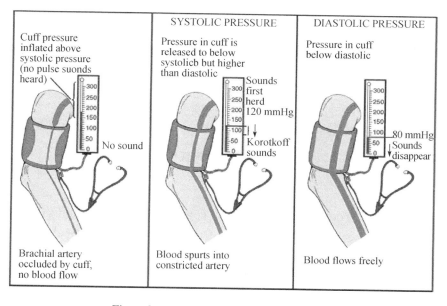

Figure 3-4　Measurement of blood pressure

(5) Observation items

① Open the switch of the sphygmomanometer, and inflate the cuff until you cannot hear the pulse sound.

② Slowly reduce the pressure in the cuff (approximately 1 to 2 mmHg per second) while listening through the stethoscope for sounds.

③ Note the pressure value at which a sharp, tapping sound is first heard. This is the systolic pressure. Continue to reduce the cuff pressure slowly, to find out the pressure at which the sound level suddenly becomes weak. This is the diastolic pressure. Some people make the pressure value at which the sound disappeared as diastolic pressure.

④ Record your measurement results: Systolic pressure/diastolic pressure mmHg (kPa.).

Notices

(1) The sounds are soft and therefore room noise must be kept to minimum.

(2) The earpiece of the stethoscope must be consistent with the direction of external auditory canal opening. To avoid the spirant influence that generates by pipe friction, we must avoid the two connecting pipes cross to each other.

(3) The tester must be quiet and relax to avoid the effects that caused by movement and mental stress.

(4) Don't tie the blood pressure cuff too tight or too loose.

(5) If you found the blood pressure is above the normal range, you should take the arm cuff off first, and measure the pressure again after a rest for at least 10 minutes.

(6) When you finish your measurement, remember to shut off the sphygmomanometer switch to avoid the leakage of the mercury.

Questions and discussions

(1) What factors can affect the arterial blood pressure measurement?

(2) Why can't you reduce the cuff pressure too fast or too slow when you measure arterial blood pressure?

(Lijuan Shi)

Experiment 8   Determination of half-life of drug plasma concentration

Experimental purpose

1. To learn how to determine the plasma concentration of sodium salicylate.

2. To grasp the method for calculation of the plasma half-life of drug.

Experimental principles

Most drugs are eliminated from the body with first-order kinetics. If the drug is eliminated by first-order process, the course of the semilogarithmic plot of plasma concentration-time curve appears linear: $\log C_t = \log C_0 - k/2.303\ t$. The plasma half-life ($t_{1/2}$) is the time it takes for the plasma concentration or the amount of drug in the body to be reduced by 50%. Calculation formula: $t_{1/2} = 0.693/k$.

Experimental materials

Instruments: surgical instruments, operation table, arterial cannula, bulldog clamp, syringes tube, tube rack, micropipettor, spectrophotometer, centrifuge, computer

Drugs: 25% urethane, 10% sodium salicylate, 10% trichloroacetic acid, 10% trichloride ferric, 1% heparin

Experimental subjects

Rabbit

Experimental procedures

1. Intubating the common carotid artery

The rabbit is weighed and administered 25% urethane (4 ml/kg) through the marginal vein in the ear. After anesthesia, the rabbit is fixed on the operation table for rabbit. Expose the common carotid artery, clamp the artery with the bulldog-clamp at the side of the heart, then make a little incision on the artery, insert the arterial cannula into the artery toward the heart, tie the cannula and artery together. 1% heparin (1 ml/kg) is administered by the marginal vein in the animal's ear to prevent the coagulation of blood.

2. Harvesting blood samples and Administering

The bulldog-clamp is loosed and blood ($\geqslant$1 ml) flows into a clean sample tube as the control; 10% Sodium salicylate (150 mg/kg, 1.5 ml/kg) is administered by the marginal vein of the animal's ear. Then harvest blood samples at 5, 15, 25, 35 and 45 min after drug administration respectively.

3. Determining the plasma concentration of sodium salicylate.

(1) Exactly draw 1 ml of blood samples with micropipettor into clean tubes, then 3.5 ml of trichloroacetic acid (10%) will be added into each tube. After mixing, samples will be centrifuged at 2,500 ~ 3,000 rpm/min for 5 mins. Then 3 ml of supernatant from each tube will be transferred into another clean tubes followed by addition of 0.3 ml of trichloride ferric (10%) into these tubes. At this moment, the purple color will appear in the tubes. Then measure the the optical density (OD) of each tube by using the spectrophotometer at 520 nm of wavelength.

(2) Exactly draw 1ml of blood samples with micropipettor into clean tubes, then 3.5 ml of trichloroacetic acid (10%) will be added into each tube. After mixing, samples will be centrifuged at 2,500 ~ 3,000 rpm/min for 5 mins. Then 3 ml of supernatant from each tube will be transferred into another clean tubes. Then measure the optical density (OD) of each tube by using the spectrophotometer at 300 nm of wavelength.

Fill in the experimental results in Table 3-7

Table 3-7　Data of the time-optical density of sodium salicylate

Time(min)	Control	After administering				
		5	15	25	30	45
Optical density						

Calculating half-life

(1) Run the RM6240 EC system in computer, select pharmacological experiment, enter into "half-life experiment"; input time and Optical density of each tube

respectively, then run "Calculate". Finally get the equation with linear regression and plasma half-life of sodium salicylate.

(2) Calculate $t_{1/2}$ according the following formula:

$$t_{1/2} = 0.301(t_2 - t_1)/\lg D_1 - \lg D_2,$$

t_1, t_2 represents times after the drug was administered, D_1 represents optical density of t_1 sample, D_2 represents optical density of t_2 sample

Notices

1. Avoid injecting drug subcutaneously.

2. Be cautious of all the procedures in this experiment, otherwise it will cause the unexpected results.

Questions and discussion

1. What is the clinical significance of determining the plasma half-life of a drug?

2. What are the characteristics of first order eliminations?

(Hua Liu)

Experiment 9　Acute intoxication of organophosphates and its treatment

Experimental purpose

Observe the toxic symptoms of organophosphates and analyze the mechanism of atropine and pralidoxime iodide (PAM) based on the antagonism action of the two drugs on organophosphates.

Experimental principles

Under the normal physiological circumstances, the constant quantity of acetylcholine in the body is maintained by acetylcholinesterase in the synaptic space. Inhibitors of acetylcholinesterase have the capacity to cause noticeable accumulation of acetylcholine in the body, which results in a series of toxic symptoms. M receptor blockers can directly antagonize various symptoms mediated by M receptors. Cholinesterase reactivating drugs are able to reactive inhibited acetylcholinesterase in a short time, so they can relieve or eliminate the toxic symptoms. As for the treatment of intoxication of organophosphates, the synergistic action of these two kinds of drugs and their difference can be analyzed through the toxic symptoms and their remission.

Experimental materials

(1) Instruments: rabbit boxes, syringes (1 ml, 5 ml, 10 ml), ruler, filter paper.

(2) Drugs: dipterex (5%, w/v), atropine sulphate (0.05%, w/v), PAM (2.5%, w/v).

Experimental subjects

Rabbit.

84

Experimental procedures

Weigh the rabbit and fix it in the rabbit boxes. Observe and record the following indices: frequency and extent of breathing, diameter of pupil, saliva secretion, excretion of urine and feces, and tremor of skeletal muscles.

Inject 75 mg/kg 5% dipterex intravenously. Observe the above-mentioned indices and record them when the toxic symptoms are obvious. Inject intravenously immediately the rabbit with 0.05% atropine sulphate 1 mg/kg (2 ml/kg). About 10 minutes later, inject intravenously the rabbit with 2.5% PAM 75 mg/kg (3 ml/kg). Then observe whether the toxic symptoms are relieved. Record the indices when the toxic symptoms are obviously relieved.

Symptom

(1) Breath: anhelation or not.

(2) Pupil: measure the diameter of pupil.

(3) Saliva secretion: observe the quantity of the saliva. " – " for no saliva; " + " for a little saliva; " + + " for moderate saliva; " + + + " for much saliva.

(4) Urine and feces: " – " for no urine or feces; " + " for a little urine or feces; " + + " for moderate urine or feces; " + + + " for much urine or feces.

(5) Tremor of muscle: " – " for no tremor of muscle; " + " for mild tremor; " + + " for moderate tremor; " + + + " for serious tremor of muscle and the rabbit cannot stand by itself.

Record the results according to Table 3-8.

Table 3-8 Indices of acute intoxication of organophosphates and its treatment in rabbit

	Breathing	Diameter of pupil	Saliva secretion	Feces excretion	Tremor of muscle
Normal					
After treated with dipterex					
After treated with atropine					
After treated with PAM					

Notices

(1) Dipterex is a powerful toxicant, and it can be absorbed via skin. If your hands touch the drug, wash your hands with water immediately. Don't use soap, dipterex can be transformed into a stronger toxicity of dichlorvos in alkaline environment.

(2) Since the size of pupil is influenced by light, the condition of the light should keep the same throughout the experiment.

(3) Observe the symptoms and timely record.

Experiment 10   Anticonvulsive effect of Barbiturates on electroconvulsive mice model

Experimental purpose

(1) To learn the method of electricity-induced convulsions

(2) To observe the anticonvulsive effects of barbiturates on mice

Experimental principles

Barbiturates have extensive inhibitory effects on central nervous system. The inhibitory effect strengthens as the dose increases, which progressively cause sedation, sleep, anticonvulsion and narcotism symptoms in experimental animals.

Experimentalmaterials

(1) Instruments: electricity stimulator, bell jar, balance, syringes, clips

(2) Drugs: 0.5% sodium phenobarbital, normal saline

Experimental subjects

Two mice (male Kun Ming strain), weighing about $18 \sim 22$ g.

Experimental procedures

(1) Adjust the stimulator, set the parameters as following:

Front Panel: Mode of stimulating = single

Stimulating time = 0.25 seconds

Frequency = $8 \sim 1$ Hz

Rear Panel: Working condition = electric shock

Voltage = 90 V

Connect AC output to two clips

(2) Hold and weigh two mice. Use one of the clips to clamp the skin between the ears of the mouse; use the other to clamp the skin of the lower mandible. Turn on the power; push the start button to give stimulation. Leave the voltage unchanged, adjust the frequency and determine the electro-convulsion threshold. Observe the behavior when the mice get electro-convulsions. Normally, the mice will experience Body Rigidity, Posterior limb straighten and Clonus. In this experiment, Posterior limb straighten is considered as the electro-convulsion sign. Once electro-convulsion threshold is determined, one of the mice receives 0.5% Phenobarbital injection (i. p.) while the other one receives normal saline (i. p.) as control. 30 mins later, stimulate these two mice with the same threshold and observe the behavior changes of these two mice respectively.

(3) Fill the experimental results in the following table 3-9.

Table 3-9 Anticonvulsive effect of sodium phenobarbital

Animal	Weight (g)	Drug	Dose (mg/kg)	Threshold Frequency (Hz)	Posterior limb straighten	
					Pre-treatment	Post-treatment
1						
2						

Notice

(1) Due to individual difference, animals may have different electro-convulsion frequency, and be aware to adjust the frequency in descending order.

(2) Make sure to use the same stimulation frequency before and after the drug treatment.

(3) Make sure the working condition of the machine in the rear panel is set on electric shock mode during the whole experiment procedure.

Questions and Discussions

What is the mechanism involved in the anti-convulsion effect of barbiturates?

(*Xinjian Zhu*)

Experiment 11 Effect of chlorpromazine on mice aggressive behavior

Experimental purpose

(1) To learn the method of inducing aggressive behavior by electricity stimulator.

(2) To observe the tranquilizing effects of chlorpromazine on mice aggressive behavior.

Experimental principles

Chlorpromazine has strong sedative effects on central nervous system, which significantly alleviate maniac state and aggressive behavior. This tranquilizing effect of chlorpromazine is also called neuroleptic effect.

Experimentalmaterials

(1) Instruments: electricity stimulator, bell jar, balance, syringes, clips

(2) Drugs: 0.05% chlorpromazine hydrochloride, normal saline

Experimental subjects

four mice (male Kun Ming strain), weighing about 18~22 g.

Experimental procedures

(1) Adjust the stimulator, set the parameters as following:

Front Panel: Mode of stimulating = Continuous B

Stimulating time = 1 seconds

Frequency = 8 Hz

Rear Panel: Working condition = electric shock

Voltage = 60~90 V

Connect AC output to stimulating box.

(2) Take four different cage housed mice, weigh and label them. Randomly pick up two of the mice as a group and put them into the electricity-stimulating box and cover them with a glass bell jar. Turn on the power and push the start button of the electricity stimulator to give stimulation. Adjust the voltage and determine the threshold for mice aggressive behavior. Observe the behavior when the mice get irritated. Generally, the mice will be regarded as irritated when they are fighting and biting each other. Once the voltage threshold for mice aggressive behavior is determined, one group of mice receive chlorpromazine hydrochloride injection (i. p.) while the other group receive normal saline (i. p.) as control. 30 mins later, stimulate these two groups of mice with the same threshold and observe the behavior changes of the mice respectively.

(3) Fill the experimental results in the following table 3-10.

Table 3-10   Effect of chlorpromazine

Animal Number	Body Weight (g)	Drug	Dose (mg/kg)	Threshold voltage (V)	Aggressive behavior	
					Pre	Post
1						
2						
3						
4						

Notice

(1) Due to individual difference, animals may have different voltage threshold of aggressive behavior, and be aware to adjust the voltage in ascending order.

(2) Make sure to use the same stimulation threshold before and after the drug treatment.

(3) Make sure the working condition of the machine in the rear panel is set on electric shock and irritating mode during the whole experiment procedure.

Questions and Discussions

What is the mechanism involved in the tranquilizing effect of chlorpromazine?

(*Xinjian Zhu*)

Experiment 12   Recording and observation of compound action potential of a nerve trunk

Experimental purpose

(1) To isolate the sciatic nerve from a toad leg.

(2) To record and observe the compound action potential (CAP) from the sciatic nerve trunk.

(3) To examine the effect of stimulus intensity on the magnitude of the CAP.

(4) To measure the conduction velocity of CAP.

Experimental principles

An action potential (AP) is a rapid change of membrane potential consisting of both depolarization and repolarization. When AP occurs, the membrane is excited. In neurons, the membrane at rest is polarized as being negative inside. When AP occurs, the polarity turns opposite tentatively: negative outside at the site of AP. The change in membrane potential can be detected by electrodes. An AP elicited at any one point on an excitable membrane usually excites adjacent portions of the membrane, resulting in propagation of the AP along the membrane. The traveling AP can go across a long distance without attenuation. Measuring the time needed for the AP to travel between the two points renders the speed of AP (the velocity = distance/time).

The sciatic nerve is the nerve trunk connecting the spinal cord with the far end of a leg. It consists of a bundle of nerve fibers. When the nerve bundle is stimulated at one point, some or all of those fibers are excited, depending on the strength of the stimuli. Their APs show difference in threshold and conduction velocity. The resulting electric signals recorded from the surface of the nerve trunk are the sum of APs produced by each individual nerve fiber (axon). Therefore, they are called compound action potentials (CAPs), which should be distinguished from the *action potentials* generated by individual fibers.

CAPs can be recorded from the extracellular surface of a nerve trunk (Fig 8-1). Usually, stimulating electrodes are applied to one end of the nerve trunk; and recording electrodes towards the other end. If the nerve is stimulated with a current pulse of sufficient amplitude, the action potentials will be produced and will propagate from the stimulating electrodes toward the recording electrodes. The aggregate effect of many action potentials is an extracellular wave of negative potential, moving along the surface of the nerve. The wave will produce a negative pulse as it passes the first recording electrode (negative for the first electrode as compared with the second one). Later, the negative wave passes the second recording electrode. At this time, the membrane potential under the first electrode is recovered (repolarized, partially at least), rending it positive as compared with the potential seen by the second electrode. If the recording electrodes are spaced appropriately, a*diphasic compound action potential* can be seen (Figure 3-5).

The propagation of AP can be blocked by a number of methods including mechanical pressure applied to the nerve or crushing the nerve with forceps. If the CAP is blocked between the two recording electrodes so that it could not reach the second recording electrode, a*monophasic compound action potential* will be recorded.

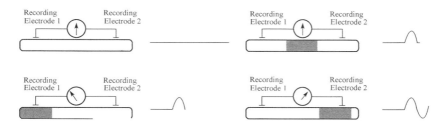

Figure 3-5　The diphasic CAP recorded by a pair of extracellular electrodes

The stimulus strength that is just enough to give a measurable response is termed as the *threshold*. Any stimulus of greater strength is a *suprathreshold one*. The strength that gives the maximal response is the *maximal stimulus*; any strength greater than this is *supramaximal*. The CAP amplitude is graded in nature, in striking contrast to the all-or-none response of a single axon.

The conduction velocity of an AP varies across different kinds of nerve fibers. The velocity is determined by several factors including the axon diameter and myelination, pH and temperature, etc. The conduction velocity (V) of sciatic nerve fibers ranges between 20 and 50 m/s. By definition, the conduction velocity of a CAP is calculated as

$$V = d/t$$

where d: the conduction distance; and t: the conduction time.

Experimental materials

(1) Instruments: RM6240-EC Multi physiological signal collecting and processing system, operating table for frogs, a set of operating tools, pithing needle, nerve chamber.

(2) Drugs: Ringer's solution

Experimental subjects

Toads

Experimental procedures

(1) Destroy the brain and the spinal cord of the toad with a pitching needle.

Pierce through the foramen magnum into the cranial cavity using the pithing needle to destroy the brain, and then reverse the needle and pierce the spinal canal to destroy the spinal cord of the toad.

(2) Cut off the toad's vertebral column above the origin of the sciatic nerve, including the viscera.

(3) Remove the skin from both legs.

Grab the vertebrae with a pair of forceps and grab a fold of skin with another pair of forceps and pull the skin down all the way towards the toes. By doing so, a naked sample of lower body trunk along with two legs is obtained.

(4) Place the sample in Ringer's solution for at least 5 min. Wash your hands and

the used apparatus. This step is necessary to clean out all the dirt and toxins from the toad skin that may influence the nerve function.

(5) Remove the urostyle.

(6) Fix the sample with pin on the dissecting table with the ventral side up.

(7) Tie off the sciatic nerve at its origin where it leaves the spinal cord with a piece of cotton thread. Free the nerve from the surrounding tissue in the abdomen using a blunt glass hook.

(8) Flip over the preparation to show the dorsal side of the legs and expose the nerve in the thigh where it lies deeply between the muscles. Cut through the overlying membranes and uncover the nerve to free the nerve down to the ankle.

(9) Tie off the nerve at the ankle end with another piece of thread. Cut the nerve just below where it is tied, and cut away any remaining branches.

(10) Gently raise the nerve by lifting the thread at both ends, and immerse the sciatic nerve in Ringer's solution for at least 5 min.

(11) Gently place the sciatic nerve over the electrodes in the nerve chamber with the thicker end of the nerve over the stimulating electrodes which are closely spaced than the recording electrodes.

(12) Run the software to stimulate the nerve and observe the trace on the screen.

Observation items

(1) Observe the biphasic action potential induced by stimulus. Identify the stimulus artifact and the action potential.

Start with a weak stimulus and gradually increase the level. The display initially will show only a brief biphasic deflection, with a duration of the stimulus impulse. This is the *stimulus artifact* (SA), which is the result of electrical leakage from the stimulating electrodes. SA marks the exact time when the nerve is shocked. Continue to gradually increase the stimulus voltage; note that the size of the SA also increases. Then, a new, small, delayed deflection appear right to the SA, this is the CAP, whose shape is also characterized as biphasic but with longer duration.

(2) Study the effect of stimulus intensity on the magnitude of the CAP. Increase the stimulus intensity gradually; when a CAP first appears, this is the threshold stimulus. Write down the intensity (threshold intensity). Continue to increase the stimulus intensity, observing the changes in shape and magnitude of the CAP until further increase in stimulus voltage no longer increases the amplitude of the CAP. This is the maximal stimulus intensity.

(3) Observe the biphasic action potential induced by the maximal stimulus. Measure the latency, amplitude, and duration of the CAP. The latency of the onset of the CAP is the time between the onset of the SA and the onset of the CAP. The amplitude of the CAP is the voltage value of the peak of the CAP response. The duration of the CAP is

the time from the beginning of the positive phase to the end of the negative phase of the CAP.

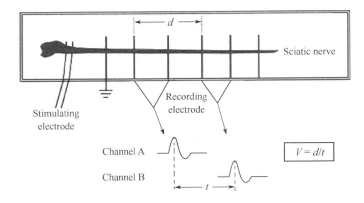

Figure 3-6 Determination of the conduction velocity of the CAP

(4) Calculate the conduction velocity of action potential. Measure the time for CAP peak travel from recording channel A to B (t) in milliseconds. Measure the distance between two recording electrodes in millimeters (d). Calculate the nerve impulse velocity (v, $v = d/t$) (Fig 3-6).

(5) Nip the nerve tightly between the two recording electrodes with tweezers. Observe the monophasic action potential. Measure the amplitude and duration of the monophasic CAP.

Notices

(1) During the dissection, try not to stretch the nerve and avoid touching the nerve with anything metal to avoid damaging the nerve.

(2) Keep the nerve moist with appropriate amount of Ringer's solution during the experiment. The nerve will malfunction if it is too dry. On the other hand, too much solution will create a short circuit between the two recording electrode, this will reduce the CAP amplitude recorded.

(3) Avoid picking up the nerve with forceps: handling should always be done by gently lifting the nerve by the attached threads. Stretching can discontinue the nerve fiber and destroy the propagation mechanisms.

Questions and discussion

(1) If the nerve trunk is replaced by a wet cotton thread, what will the results be?

(2) In the experiment, how can you distinguish between the stimulus artifact and the real CAP?

(3) What is the difference between the action potential of a single axon and the compound action potential?

(*Lijie Liu*)

92

Experiment 13 Analysis of edema related factors

Experimental purpose

To replicate the animal model of edema, and to observe the effects of capillary hydrostatic pressure and colloid osmotic pressure in blood vessel on the formation of edema.

Experimental principles

By using circulatory system of a toad, different liquid with certain property is quantitatively perfused into the aortic arch, and the liquid flowing out mainly from the hepatic vein is collected at the same time. Compare the amount of outflow fluid with that of inflow fluid, and the difference between these two amounts can reflect whether the accumulation of fluid in the body.

Experimental materials

(1) Instruments: surgical instruments, perfusion device, cylindrical glass (10 ml), beaker (50 ml, 5 ml), dropper, syringe (1 ml).

(2) Drugs: 1% heparin, ringer solution, dextran-40 solution.

Experimentalsubjects

Toad

Experimental procedures

(1) Prepare the toad blood vessel perfusion device. Connect an empty syringe barrel (20 ml) to one end of a segment of infusion catheter with a water stop clamp on it. Meanwhile, connect the joint of a syringe needle with a fine plastic tube to another end of the catheter. Set the empty syringe barrel on the iron support platform. At about 30 cm distance to the syringe barrel nipple, fix an iron clamp to support a special toad board. Fill the perfusion device with Ringer solution and remove gas bubbles from the tube system and clamp the catheter.

(2) Animal treatment. Destroy the brain and spinal cord of the toad using a metal explorer and put the dead toad on the board. Open the peritoneal cavity by cutting the abdominal wall with a scissors along 0.5 cm left to the abdominal median line. Inject 0.1 ml of heparin into the vena epigastrica for preventing blood clotting. Extend the opening of the pleural cavity by cutting the thoracic wall and the sternoclavicular joint. Both the up and lower sides of the opening have to be extended to the bilateral vertebral column, to prevent the fluid accumulation in the cavities. Cut the pericardium with an ophthalmic scissors and expose the heart.

(3) Perfusion experiments with toad blood vessel. Lift the liver up and expose the vena cava posterior. Put a piece of thread behind the vein to block local blood return. Put two pieces of thread behind the aortic bow. One of them is used to ligate the isolated artery at its proximal part. Cut the aortic bow with the ophthalmic scissors and insert a

thin plastic tube filled with Ringer solution into the artery and fix it with the other one of thread. Cut the hepatic vein to let the fluid flow out. Slope the board on perfusion device and adjust the speed of perfusion by waterstop clamp to 25~30 drops per minute. Then, do the following experiment:

① When the surface of inflow fluid in the syringe barrel is down to the baseline, pour 10 ml of Ringer solution into the barrel, and collect the outflow fluid from one side of the board at once until the surface is down to the baseline again. Record the outflow volume and repeat the above procedures one more time.

② Pour 10 ml of Dextran-40 solution into the syringe barrel and collect the outflow fluid with a beaker until the surface is at the baseline, then record outflow volume and repeat the procedure one more time.

③ Pour 10 ml of Ringer solution into the syringe barrel and ligate vena cava posterior. Collect the outflow fluid until the surface is down to the baseline. Record the volume and repeat the test.

(4) Record the results in table 3-11.

Table 3-11　Effects of different factors on circulatory perfusion of toad

Factor		1	2	3	4	5	6	7	8
Ringer solution 10 ml	First time								
	Second time								
Dextran-40 solution 10 ml	First time								
	Second time								
Ringer solution 10 ml + Vein ligation	First time								
	Second time								

Notices

(1) Thoroughly expose peritoneal and pleural cavities to prevent the fluid from accumulating in these cavities.

(2) A baseline should be marked on the syringe barrel nipple which is about 30 cm from the toad board. Each time when the surface of inflow fluid in the syringe barrel is down to the baseline, pour new prepared inflow fluid into the barrel immediately. Make sure to slope the board on perfusion device, let the outflow fluid be collected in one direction.

(3) Fill the perfusion device with Ringer solution to remove gas bubbles in order to avoid the air embolism in the body of toad.

(4) Heparinized circulation can keep patency for sustained perfusion.

(5) Ligate the isolated aortic bow at its proximal to the heart with a piece of thread and keep the ends of the thread for traction. Put another piece of thread through the aortic bow at its distal to the heart. Cut a small hole on the aortic bow with an ophthalmic scissors and insert a thin plastic catheter filled with Ringer solution into the

artery, and fix the catheter with the thread at the distal part of the artery. Avoid *puncturing the artery*.

(6) The speed of infusion should be timely adjusted by the waterstop clamp due to different viscosity of inflow fluids.

(7) The cylindrical glass should be washed with clean water in before taking the exact amount of each inflow fluid.

Questions and discussion

(1) What can be observed on the amount of outflow fluid when perfusion with Ringer solution? Why?

(2) What can be observed on the amount of outflow fluid when perfusion with Dextran-40 solution? Why?

(3) What can be observed on the amount of outflow fluid when perfusion with Ringer solution following ligation of the vena cava posterior? Why?

(Wei Zhang and Weiping Yu)

Experiment 14   Hypoxia

Experimental purpose

(1) To know the classification of hypoxia and to replicate the animal models of hypotonic and hemic hypoxia.

(2) To observe the changes including breath, color of skin and mucous membrane, animal activity in each model of different types of hypoxia.

Experimental principles

(1) Replicate the animal model of hypotonic hypoxia by suffocation.

(2) Replicate the animal models of hemic hypoxia by carbon monoxide poisoning or nitrite poisoning.

Experimental materials

(1) Instruments: wide-mouthed bottles (125 ml), dropper, syringe (1 ml), double concave slide, and scissors

(2) Drugs: CO gas, 10% sodium hydroxide, 1% sodium nitrite, 0.5% methylthioninium chloride.

Experimentalsubjects

Mice.

Experimental procedures

1. Hypotonic hypoxia

(1) Take two mice with an approximated body weight (BW) and put them into two uncovered wide-mouthed bottle (125 ml), respectively and observe the color of ears, tail, mouth and oral lips, the respiratory frequency (R. F. , times/10 seconds × 6).

(2) Closely cover one bottle and record the time, while the other one keep open as

control. Observe the above mentioned indexes every 3 minutes.

(3) Record the dead time of the mouse in the covered bottle and execute the control mouse by spinal cord disjunction. Dissect two mice and observe the color of blood and internal organs. Keep the dead bodies of mice for comparison with others at last.

2. Hemic hypoxia

(1) Poisoned by CO

① Take three mice with an approximated BW and observe the color of ears, tail, mouth and oral lips, as well as R. F. (times/10 seconds × 6).

② One mouse is poisoned by 15 ml CO to death. Then dissect the mouse and observe the color of blood and internal organs. Keep the dead body for comparison with others at last.

③ Another one mouse is poisoned by 15 ml CO to twitch. Then immediately remove the mouse from the bottle to rescue it. Observe the changes of above indexes and its survival situation. Execute it by spinal cord disjunction if it is still survival.

④ Put the third mouse into a bottle and closely cover the bottle at the same time as the bottles containing the mice poisoned by CO are covered. As a control, release it when the other two mice poisoned by CO to death or to be rescued. Execute it by spinal cord disjunction at last.

Appendix: Qualitative test of carbon monoxide (sodium hyfroxide method): 2 drops of 10% NaOH were dripped into each of two grooves of the double concave slide, then add one drop of blood from the carbon monoxide poisoned mouse or from the control mouse into each groove of the side, respectively, and mixed them well. Blood containing carbon monoxide can remain pink for a few minutes, while blood without carbon monoxide immediately turns brown.

(2) Poisoned by nitrite.

① Take two mice with an approximated BW and observe the color of ears, tail, mouth and oral lips, as well as R. F. (times/10 seconds × 6).

② One mouse is intraperitoneally injected (I. P.) with 1 ml of 1% sodium nitrite. Record the injection time, and observe R. F. and the color of ears, tail, mouth and oral lips every 2 minutes until the animal dies. Then dissect the mouse and observe the color of blood and internal organs. Keep the dead body for comparison with others at last.

③ The other one mouse is I. P. with 1 ml of 1% sodium nitrite, 5 minutes later treated by intraperitoneal injection of 0. 4 ml of 0. 5% methylthioninium Chloride. Observe the changes of above indexes and its survival situation. Execute it by spinal cord disjunction if it is still survival. Dissect the mouse and observe the color of its blood and internal organs.

Detoxification mechanism of Methylene Blue (MB):

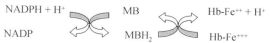

96

3. Record the results in table 3-12.

Table 3-12　Changes of breath and tissue color in different types of hypoxic mice

Model	R. F. (times/min)	Tissue colour		
		Skin	Blood	Internal organs
Control				
Suffocation				
Poisoned by nitrite				
Poisoned by CO				

Notices

(1) Closely cover the bottle when replicate the animal model of hypotonic hypoxia.

(2) The syringe used for each drug should be specific. Pay attention to the dosage of each drug used.

(3) Each mouse should be marked. Rescue the indicatedanimal model in time.

(4) Take the blood of both CO poisoning mouse and control mouse at the same time while doing qualitative test of carbon monoxide.

Questions and discussion

(1) What are the colors of skin and mucous membrane in hypotonic and hemic hypoxia?

(2) What are the mechanisms underlying the changes of breath and tissue color in different types of hypoxia according to the experimental results.

(3) What is cyanosis? In which types of hypoxia can cyanosis be found?

(*Kai Liao and Weiping Yu*)

Experiment 15　Regulation of respiration

Experimental purpose

(1) To learn the method of recording respiratory movements in rabbit.

(2) To observe the effects of some regulating factors on respiratory movements and analyze the mechanism of their actions.

Experimental principles

Respiratory movement is controlled by rhythmic activity of the respiratory center. Respiratory depth and frequency are altered by the changes in both internal and external environments, which modulate the respiratory movement via the nervous system to meet the body's need under different environments. There are many regulating mechanisms involving the respiratory nervous center, which modulate the respiration movement through pulmonary stretch reflex, chemical control of breathing, respiratory muscle proprioceptive reflex, and so on. The major environmental factors include P_{O2}, P_{CO2} and hydrogen-ion concentration: respiration will increase when arterial P_{O2} decreases, P_{CO2} and hydrogen-ion concentration increase.

Experimental materials

(1) Instruments: RM6240 EC Multi-physiological signal collecting and processing system, a suit of surgical instruments a rabbit's operation table, trachea cannula, syringe (20 ml), syringe(2 ml), rubber tube (30 cm), a bag of carbon dioxide, tension transducer

(2) Drugs: 25% urethane, 3% lactic acid, normal saline.

Experimental subjects

Rabbit.

Experimental procedures

(1) Handling, weighing, anesthesia and fixing rabbit (refer instruction for Experiment 1).

(2) Operation in neck for endotracheal intubation (refer Experiment 1)

Separate the right and left vagus nerve in the carotid sheath: Use glass needles to separate the vagus nerve and place a piece of silk thread under each nerve (as shown in the figure 3-7 below).

(3) Separate small diaphragm muscle: Find xiphoid process with your index finger. Open the upper abdomen about 2 cm incision along linea alba above the xiphoid process, then expose the xiphoid process. Cut the peritoneum rounding xiphoid process, insert a Tissue Clamp under the sternum body. Then separate the small diaphragm muscle from the sternum body, cut at the conjunct point of sternum body and xiphoid process. Lastly pinch through the xiphoid process with a small hook (as shown in the figure 3-8 below).

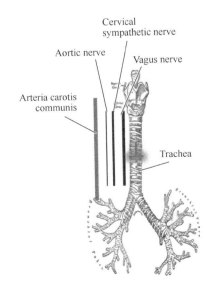

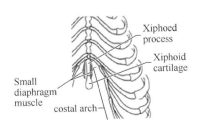

Figure 3-7　Diagram of carotid sheath and trachea　　　Figure 3-8　Diagram of small diaphragm muscle.

(4) Hardware connection: Use a thread to connect the hook with tension transducer as shown in the Figure 3-9 below. The diaphragm muscle is connected with tension transducer and the output end of the transducer is connected to the recording system.

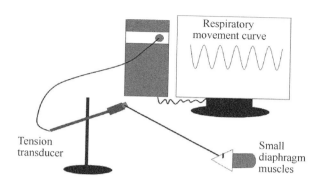

Figure 3-9   Connection of RM6240 EC system with small diaphragm muscle

Recording: record the respiratory movement with the RM6240 EC Multi-physiological signal collecting and processing system

Items for observations

(1) Record normal respiratory movement curve for one minute.

(2) Increase CO_2 concentration in the inspiratory air with CO_2 gasbag, and observe the change of the respiratory curve, and analyze the mechanism of CO_2 actions.

(3) Increase dead space by connecting 30cm rubber tube with endotrachealintubation and observe the change of the respiratory curve, and analyze the mechanism of its actions.

(4) Increase airway resistance by clamping 1/2 – 2/3 rubber tube of endotrachealintubation and observe the change of respiratory movement curve, and analyze the mechanism of its actions.

(5) Inject 3% lactic acid (1 ml/kg) into the marginal ear vein and observe the change of the respiratory curve, and analyze the mechanism of its actions.

(6) Observe pulmonary stretch reflex phenomena and analyze it. Inject 20ml air into the rabbit's lung at the end of inspiration, then hold 5~10 s, remove the syringe. When rabbit's respiratory movement curve recovers to normal state, draw 20 ml air from rabbit's lung at the end of expiration, then hold 5~10 s, remove the syringe.

(7) Cut off right and left vagus nerves, and observe the changes of respiratory movement curve.

(8) Then repeat the 6th process. Observe the changes of the respiratory curve.

(9) Save the file when you finish the experiment.

(10) Fill the experimental results in the Table 3-13.

Table 3-13   Effects of different factors on frequency and amplitude of respiration

Items		Frequency (breaths/min)	Amplitude(cm)
Control		normal	normal
CO_2			
Dead space			
Airway resistance			
lactic acid			
Pulmonary stretch reflex	Pulmonary inflation reflex		
	Pulmonary deflation reflex		
Cut two Vagus nerves			
Cut two Vagus nerves	Pulmonary inflation reflex		
	Pulmonary deflation reflex		

Notices

(1) To avoid damages to small diaphragm muscle, a mosque forceps must be used to gently separate muscle from the sternum body. Don't cut the peritoneum too deep at the conjunct point between costal margin and sternum body. This will avoid the formation of pneumothorax and large bleeding.

(2) To avoid fatigue of the small diaphragm muscle, the connecting string must be vertical with the plane of tension transducer for the most effective pulling. Additionally, don't move this connecting string in any way during the experiment. Otherwise, the respiratory movement curve is corrupted and the comparison across different manipulations would be invalid.

(3) The upper abdominal incision should not be too long (approximately 2 cm is good). Otherwise, abdominal organs may bulge out and affect the movement of the small diaphragm muscle.

Questions and discussion

(1) Across regulating factors observed (CO_2, lactic acid and dead space), which one is most important for respiratory stimulation, why?

(2) If the carotid body is narcotized first, what are the expected effect of inhaling high concentration CO_2 and intravenous injection of lactic acid? Why?

(3) Based upon the results of experimental items 6, 7, and 8, describe the strategies of scientific research.

(Qingying Xun)

Experiment 16   The factors affecting urine formation

Experiment purposes

To learn how to collect urine from bladder in rabbits and to observe the effects of different factors on final urine production

Experiment principles

The process of urine production includes filtration of glomerular, absorption and secretion of renal tubule and collecting duct. The motive power of glomerular filtration is glomerular effective filtration pressure, while glomerular capillary blood pressure, plasma colloid osmotic pressure and the renal capsular pressure can affect glomerular filtration pressure. Therefore, the factors affecting above-mentioned pressure will finally influence renal infiltration function. In addition, the solute concentration in renal tubule and the antidiuretic hormone are also important factors that affect reabsorption and secretion function of renal tubule and collecting duct. From the above, all of these factors can regulate the production of final urine.

Experiment materials

(1) Instruments: RM6240 EC Multi-physiological signal collecting and processing system, operation table for rabbit, surgical instruments for mammals, endotracheal intubation, arterial cannula, bladder intubation, blood pressure transducer, drop recorder, culture dish.

(2) Drugs: 25% urethane, 25% glucose, heparin, 1 : 10,000 norepinephrine solution, furosemide and pituitrin.

Experiment subjects

Rabbits

Experiment procedures

1. Operation

(1) Hold a rabbit and get the weight.

(2) Inject 25% (4 ml/kg) urethane through rabbit's ear marginal vein for anesthesia, and fix the animal on the operating table with supine position. After that, keep the venous unobstructed.

(3) Shear the hair on the neck and make a longitudinal incision along the middle line of the rabbit's neck. Subsequently, separate subcutaneous tissue step by step and bluntly separate muscle, so that the trachea can be exposure. Then insert the endotracheal intubation and keep rabbit breath smoothly. The surgical operation on the neck is temporarily over, cover the surgical wound with when gauze dipped in saline before.

(4) Shear the hair on the rabbit abdominal, and make a 3~5 cm incision on the right above of pubic symphysis. Open the abdominal cavity along the linea alba, expose the bladder and move the bladder out. Make a 1cm incision on the top of the bladder and insert the bladder intubation. Make sure that the intubation end is at the exit of ureter in bladder (NOT close too much to bladder wall, avoid blocking the ureter). Ligature the incision twice to fix the bladder incision on the intubation wall. After operation on abdomen, cover the gauze pre-infiltrated with saline on the surgical wound.

(5) Isolate the vagus nerve on the right side of rabbit neck.

(6) Isolate the left common carotid artery. Inject heparin solution from marginal ear vein for systemic heparinization, and fill the artery cannula with heparin solution for local heparinization. Then insert the artery cannula into the common carotid artery. After operation on the neck, connect the artery cannula with blood pressure transducer. DON'T cover the pipe of endotracheal intubation.

2. The connection and use of experimental device

Connect the blood pressure transducer to the 3rd channel of RM6240 EC Multi-physiological signal collecting and processing system and correctly record the rabbit's blood pressure. Let the urine drop from the bladder intubation onto the recorder, and connect the drop recorder to the 4th channel of RM6240 EC system. At last, connect the stimulus electrode to stimulus output channel of RM6240 EC system.

Observation items

(1) Open the bulldog clamp on carotid artery and the spring clap of balder intubation, record normal blood pressure and urine volume of rabbits.

(2) Quickly inject 20 ml saline through marginal ear vein, observe and record blood pressure and urine volume.

(3) Quickly inject 0. 3 ml 1 : 10000 norepinephrine through marginal ear vein, observe and record blood pressure and urine volume.

(4) Quickly inject 5 ml 25% glucose solution through marginal ear vein, observe and record blood pressure and urine volume.

(5) Stimulate the nerve moderately (Stimulus parameters: Intensity: $5 \sim 10$ V Width: 2 ms; Duration: $5 \sim 10$ s), then observe and record blood pressure and urine volume.

(6) Inject furosemide (5 mg/kg) through marginal ear vein, observe and record blood pressure and urine volume.

(7) Inject pituitrin (2U) through marginal ear vein, observe and record blood pressure and urine volume.

Notices

(1) To ensure the animal has enough urine in the experiment, animals should be feed with cabbage leaves before experiment or injected 40 ml saline into abdomen during the surgical operation.

(2) The surgical operation should be tender and careful, and the incision on abdomen should not be too big.

(3) Keep the marginal ear vein unobstructed, because in the experiment we need inject many times through the marginal ear vein. So when injection, start as far as possible from distal end of ear vein.

(4) Every observation item should begin only after last action is disappeared and blood pressure and urine volume recover to almost normal level, which avoid mutual interference of different factors, and also is helpful to know the drug latency period,

maximal effect and the duration time.

(5) The vagus nerve should not be over-stimulated, avoiding blood pressure drop sharply or even cardiac arrest, so the stimulation time should not be too long and the intensity not be too high.

Question and discussion

"when systemic arterial blood pressure is elevated, the urine must be increased; While the systemic arterial blood pressure is reduced, the urine must be decreased." Is that right? Why?

(Jian Yang)

Experiment 17　Effects of furosemide and hypertonic glucose on urinary excretion

Experimental purpose

To observe effects of furosemide and hypertonic glucose on excretion of water, Na^+, K^+ and Cl^-. To learn the methods of detecting potency of diuretics.

Experimental principles

Loop diuretics furosemide inhibit the luminal $Na^+/K^+/2Cl^-$ transporter in the thick ascending limb (TAL) of Henle's loop. By inhibiting this transporter, the loop diuretics reduce the reabsorption of NaCl and also diminish the lumen-positive potential that comes from K^+ recycling. This positive potential normally drives divalent cation reabsorption in the TAL, and by reducing this potential, loop diuretics cause an increase in Mg^{2+} and Ca^{2+} excretion. The proximal tubule and descending limb of Henle's loop are freely permeable to water. Any osmotically active agent that is filtered by the glomerulus is not reabsorbed which therefore causes water to be retained in these segments and promotes a water diuresis. Such agents can be used to reduce intracranial pressure and to promote prompt removal of renal toxins.

Experimental materials

Instruments: pairs of scissors (curved, straight), hemostat, eye scissors, eye tweezers, pinhead, porcelain-cup, gauze, thick rope, fine rope, urocystic cannula, syringes (5ml, 10ml, 1ml), evaporating dish, flame photometer, burette.

Drugs: normal saline, 25% urethane, 1% furosemide, 50% glucose solution, 20% chromate potassium, standard solution of argent nitrate.

Experimental subjects

Rabbit.

Experimental Procedures

1. Animal Preparation

Take a rabbit, weight it and place it into a rabbit box. Then intragastrically administer the rabbit with warm water (50 ml/kg). After 20 min, 25% urethane is injected through the marginal vein in the ear. The velocity of injection should be slow and we should monitor the respiration of the animal (about 5min). After anesthesia, the rabbit is fixed on the operating table.

2. Lower belly operation

Shear off the hair from the lower belly. Incise the skin above the public symphysis about 4 cm. Then cut the muscle at the middle of abdominal wall. Then open the abdominal cavity and expose the bladder. Take the bladder out from the abdominal cavity and put it on a piece of gauze soaked with water. Raise the two sides of the bladder at the vessel part with two hemostats. Cut a hole at the summit of the bladder. Then draw 3~4 ml urine with a clean syringe, then insert the bladder cannula into the bladder and tie the bladder cannula tightly. The gab of the bladder cannula must be toward the gab of the ureter.

3. Harvesting samples

Collect urine and record the volume every 5 min after administration, transfer the urine of 30 min into a clean glass bottle and label it "No. 1". This is the control sample. 5 mg/kg furosemide or 5 ml/kg 50% glucose is injected through the marginal vein in the ear. Collect urine and record the volume every 5 min after administration, transfer the urine of 30 min into another glass bottle and label it "No. 2".

4. Detecting concentration of Na^+ and K^+ in urine

Take 0. 2 ml of urine from No. 1 and No. 2 bottle respectively, dilute it with distilled water to 30 ml (150 times). Detect the concentration of Na^+ and K^+ in urine by flame photometer respectively. The following formula can be used to calculate the concentration of Na^+ and K^+. Na^+ (or K^+) concentration of the urine sample $C_x = A_x \times$ diluting multiple (150). A_x: reading of radian intensity of urine diluted. Calculate total amount of Na^+ and K^+ 30 min before and after administration according to the following equation respectively. Total amount of ion = ion concentration $C_x \times$ total volume of urine (ml) in 30 min.

5. Detecting concentration of Cl^- in urine

Silver ion in urine is precipitated to silver chloride by silver nitrate reagent. If silver nitrate is slightly excessive, it will react with potassium chromates to form silver chromate which appears citrus red in color. The reaction formula is as the following:

$$NaCl + AgNO_3 \rightarrow AgCl \downarrow + NaNO_3$$
$$2AgNO_3 + K_2CrO_4 \rightarrow Ag_2CrO_4 \downarrow + 2 KNO_3$$

Wash the evaporating dish with distilled water. Take 1 ml of urine from No. 1, No. 2 and No. 3 bottle respectively, dilute it with distilled water to 10 ml in a clean evaporating dish, and add two drops of chromate potassium (20%). Then slowly drop argent nitrate ($AgNO_3$) standard solution (1 ml amount to 0. 606 mg chloride ion) into the beaker, and mix thoroughly at the same time, until a stable citrus red color occurs, record the volume of used argent nitrate solution. Calculate chloride ion concentration in the urine and the total amount of chloride ion in 30 min before and after administration according to following equations respectively.

Chloridion concentration in urine (mg/ml) = the volume of used argent nitrate solution (ml) × 0.606 mg/ml ÷ 1 ml. Total amount of chloridion = chloridion concentration in urine × total volume of urine. Fill the experimental results in the Table 3-14 and 3-15

Table 3-14　Effects of different drugs on the volume of urine

Drugs	Volume of urine in 30 min (ml)	Volume of urine in every 5min(ml)					
		0~5 (min)	5~10 (min)	10~15 (min)	15~20 (min)	20~25 (min)	25~30 (min)
Control							
Furosemide (or 50% Glucose)							

Table 3-15　Effects of different drugs on Na^+, K^+ and Cl^- excretion

Drugs	Volume of urine in 30 min(ml)	Na^+		K^+		Cl^-		
		Concen -tration ($\mu g/ml$)	Total amount (mg)	Concen -tration ($\mu g/ml$)	Total amount (mg)	Volume of $AgNO_3$	Concen -tration (mg/ml)	Total amount (mg)
Control								
Furosemide (or 50% Glucose)								

Notices

1. Avoid tying the ureters to the cannula.

2. The volume of urine output must return to normal before the next step of the experiment is performed.

Questions and discussion

1. What are the definitions of diuretics and dehydration?

2. Analyze the mechanisms of urine formation and compare the different effect of Furosemide and 50% glucose.

(*Hongwei Yi*)

Experiment 18　Role of Ammonia in the Pathogenesis of Hepatic Encephlopathy

Experimental purpose

Investigate the pathogenesis and treatment of hepatic encephalopathy after creation of animal model of acute hepatic failure.

Experimental principles

(1) Ligate hepatic pedicle to make liver disablement in situ

(2) Inject preparations which containing NH_4^+, elevated concentration of blood ammonia (NH_3)

(3) Intravenous inject sodium glutamate to rescue

Experimental materials

(1) Instruments: operating table for rabbit, a set of instruments for rabbit's abdominal operation, syringe (5 ml), syringe (20 ml), syringe (50 ml), catheter.

(2) Drugs: 1% lidocaine solution: 1 bottle; 2.5% NH_4Cl application solution: 1 bottle; the solution contains 5% glucose, 2.5 g NH_4Cl and 1.5 g $NaHCO_3$; 2.5% sodium L-glutamate application solution: 1 bottle. the solution contains 5% glucose and 2.5 g sodium L-glutamate.

Experimental subjects

Rabbits.

Experimental procedures

1. Experimental rabbit

(1) Take and weigh a rabbit. Fix it supinely on an operating table. Cut off the fur from its upper abdomen. Use lidocaine solution to local infiltration anaesthesia 1 cm along the inferior extremity of the costal arch. Insert scalp needle into the marginal ear vein for later use.

(2) Cut the skin 1 cm below the xiphoid; make an archy incision paralleling the costal arch for about 8 cm and open abdominal cavity. Fasten any bleeding vessel during the process.

(3) Press the liver down and cut off the falciform ligament between the liver and the diaphragm. Turn the liver upwards and cut off the hepatogastric ligament.

(4) Find the duodenum. Avoid any blood vessels on it and make a purse-string suture with a diameter of about 1 cm. Make a small incision with the ophthalmic scissors in the center of the suture and insert the catheter about 3 cm into the jejunum. Fasten the catheter via tightening the string of the suture.

(5) Ligate the root of the left lateral lobe, left medial lobe, right medial lobe and quadrate lobe of the liver with a thick rope to completely block the blood vessel of the hepatic lobes mentioned above. Put the liver, intestines and other organs into the

abdominal cavity. Close the cavity by using cutaneous clamps.

(6) Observe and record the corneal reflex and muscle tension of the rabbit as well as its pain response to pinprick stimuli in the table below.

(7) First, carefully and slowly inject 10 ml of the NH_4Cl application solution via catheter to the duodenum in $2 \sim 3$ minutes. Subsequently, administer 5 ml of the solution every 5 minutes. Observe and record the corneal reflex and muscle tension of the rabbit as well as its pain response to pinprick stimuli. Stop the injection immediately once muscular twitch (not scrabble!) occurs. Write down the amount of the NH_4Cl application solution used. Calculate the amount per kilogram of body weight in order to compare with the control rabbit below.

(8) Treat the rabbit by injecting 30 ml of the sodium L-glutamate application solution per kilogram of body weight via the marginal ear vein. Observe and record the change in the above observation items.

2. Control rabbit

Perform the above procedures to the control rabbit except ligation of the liver in item 5. Observe the corneal reflex and muscle tension of the rabbit as well as its pain response to pinprick stimuli. Write down the amount of the NH_4Cl application solution once muscular twitch happens to control rabbit. Calculate the amount per kilogram of body weight in order to compare with the experimental rabbit.

Table 3-16 Role of ammonium in hepatic encephalopathy

Injection	Control Rabbit				Experimental Rabbit			
	Corneal Reflex	Muscle tension	Pinprick response	Muscular twitch	Corneal Reflex	Muscle tension	Pinprick response	Muscular twitch
NH_4Cl solution								
0								
10								
15								
20								
25								
30								
35								
40								
45								
50								
55								
60								
Sodium L-glutamate solution(30 ml/kg)								

The amount of NH_4Cl per kilogram of Bw

Notices

(1) The animal must be weighed first and then fixed.

(2) Local anesthetics are used for the animal to avoid struggling. Cut the abdomen gently and don't cut the liver to prevent causing hemorrhagic shock.

(3) When the operating in the upper abdomen, care should be taken to prevent massive bleeding.

(4) After the purse-string suture, put the needle on the holder.

(5) Pay attention to keep the drug away from the salvage pathway (ear vein).

(6) The catheter is inserted in the direction of jejunum, don't insert in the opposite direction.

Questions and discussion

(1) In this experiment, after ligating hepatic pedicle of the rabbit, why can the injection of NH_4Cl application solution via the duodenum cause encephalopathy?

(2) In this experiment, why can the injection of NH_4Cl application solution via the duodenum also cause encephalopathy in the control rabbit whose hepatic pedicle is not ligated?

(3) Why can the application of glutamate treat hepatic encephalopathy?

(*Kai Liao and Chuanlu Shen*)

Experiment 19   Regulation of rabbit cardiovascular activity

Experimental purpose

(1) To master the method to measure and record the arterial blood pressure in mammals.

(2) To observe the changes of arterial blood pressure and analysis the effects of nervous and humoral regulating factors on cardiovascular activity.

Experimental principles

In physiological state, the arterial blood pressures of mammals are relatively stable, which are realized through neural and humoral regulation, especially the carotid sinus-aortic arch baroreceptor reflex (Figure 3-10).

(1) Neural regulation of arterial blood pressure (carotid sinus-aortic arch baroreceptor reflex): The reflex not only lowers blood pressure when blood pressure rises, but also raises the blood pressure when blood pressure decreases. The afferent nerve of this reflex is the aortic nerve and the sinus nerve. The aorta nerve in rabbit is also called depressor nerve.

(2) Humoral regulation of arterial blood pressure: epinephrine(E), norepinephrine (NE) and acetylcholine (Ach) regulate blood pressure.

E: binding to α and β receptor to lead to an increase of cardiac output.

NE: binding to α receptor to lead to an increase of blood flow resistance.

Ach: binding to M-receptor to lead to a decrease of cardiac output.

The blood pressure is turn into an electric signal by a blood pressure transducer in the experiment, and then the signal is imported into the computer.

Experimental materials

(1) Instruments: RM6240 EC Multi-physiological signal collecting and processing system, a suit of surgical instruments, rabbit's operation table, trachea cannula, syringes (20 ml, 2 ml), scalp needle, artery tube, concave clamp, blood pressure transducer, glass dissecting, colored silk thread, thick rope

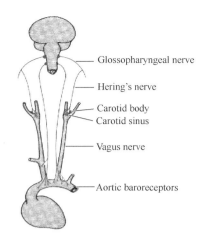

Figure 3-10　The baroreceptor system.

(2) Drugs: normal saline, 25% urethane, 1%heparin solution, 0.01% epinephrine, 0.01% norepinephrine , 0.01% acetylcholine.

Experimental subjects

Rabbit.

Experimental procedures

(1) Weighing, anesthesia and fixation (refer instruction for Experiment 1).

(2) Operation in the neck (refer instruction for Experiment 1).

① Endotracheal intubation.

② Separate the Right Depressor Nerve, the Right Vagus Nerve, the Right Common Carotid Artery.

③ Intubation in the Left Common Carotid Artery.

(3) Connect the cannula of artery to the blood pressure transducer,and remove the artery clamp. Then record the corves of arterial blood pressure with the computer.

Observation items

(1) Record normal curves of the arterial blood pressure. Identify the first level wave (heart beat wave) and the second level wave (respiratory wave). The first level wave is fluctuations of the blood pressure caused by constriction and diastole of the heart. The second level wave is fluctuations of blood pressure caused by the dilatation and shrink of the lung in respiratory.

(2) Nip closely the right common carotid artery with a carotid clamp about 5~10 seconds. Observe the change of arterial blood pressure.

(3) Stimulate the right depressor nerve with electrical stimulator (the stimulation intensity is 3~5 V, the frequency is 10~200 Hz, the wave breadth is 5 ms, and stimulation duration is 5~10 seconds). Observe the change of arterial blood pressure.

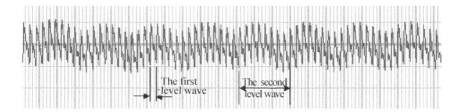

Figure 3-11　Normal curves of the arterial blood pressure

(4) Stimulate the right vagus nerve with electrical stimulator (as above). Observe the change of arterial blood pressure.

(5) Inject 0. 01% epinephrine 0. 3 ml into the ear marginal vein. Observe the change of arterial blood pressure.

(6) Inject 0. 01% norepinephrine 0. 3 ml into the ear marginal vein. Observe the change of arterial blood pressure.

(7) Inject 0. 01% acetylcholine 0. 3 ml into the ear marginal vein. Observe the change of arterial bloodpressure .

Notices

(1) Master anesthetic techniques to avoid overdose of anesthesia.

(2) Keep the arterial cannula and the common carotid artery in parallelism to avoid the artery be destroyed.

(3) Don't carry out the next item until the blood pressure restores to normal level.

(4) After each injection of drugs, immediately inject 0. 5 ml saline to prevent residual drugs in needles or local veins disturbing the action of other drugs.

Questions and discussion

(1) What is the effect on blood pressure when clamping the common carotid artery for a short time? Why? If the clamping location is above the carotid sinus, are the effects the same?

(2) What is the result of stimulating the vagus nerve? Why?

(*Yusi Cheng*)

Experiment 20　Haemodynamic effects of drugs in treating acute heart failure of rabbits

Experimental purpose

(1) To grasp the real-time measurement of hemodynamic parameters and the method of establishment of heart failure animal model.

(2) To observe the haemodynamic effects of drugs in treating acute heart failure.

Experimental principles

Heart failure (HF), is often called congestive heart failure (CHF) or congestive cardiac failure (CCF). HF is a condition in which the heart is unable to provide sufficient blood flow to meet the body's needs on condition that blood volume is normal. HF leads to inadequate organ perfusion and systemic and pulmonary volume expansion. The condition is diagnosed by patient physical examination and confirmed with echocardiography.

Clinical symptoms of CHF include: fatigue, tachycardia, decreased exercise capacity, dyspnea on exertion, cyanosis, hypotension, lower limb swelling, ascites, hepatosplenomegaly, jugular venous engorgement, pulmonary rales and orthopnea.

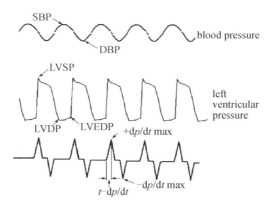

Figure 3-12   Schematic diagram of waveforms of arterial pressure and ventricular pressure

If LVEF(Left Ventricular Ejection Fractions)<40% (echocardiography) , HF may take place. BNP (B-type natriuretic peptide)>400 ng/L, or NT-proBNP (BNP with a 76 amino acid N-terminal fragment)>1500 ng/L, HF may be diagnosed.

Hemodynamic parameters:

  HR: heart rate

  SBP: systolic arterial blood pressures

  DBP: diastolic arterial blood pressures

  MAP: mean arterial blood pressures = DBP+(SBP-DBP)/3

Systolic function index:

  LVSP: left ventricular systolic pressure

  +dp/dt max: maximal increasing velocity of left ventricular pressure

  t-dp/dt max: the duration from contraction to +dp/dt max of left ventricular

Diastolic function index:

  LVDP: left ventricular diastolic pressure

  LVEDP: left ventricular end-diastolic pressure

  -dp/dt max: maximal decreasing velocity of left ventricular pressure

Experimental materials

(1) Instruments: RM6240 EC Multi-physiological signal collecting and processing

system, operating table, a set of surgical instruments, surgical scissors, operating scalpel, hemostatic forceps, artery clamp, tweezer, pincette, syringe, rope, cord, thread and et al.

(2) Drugs: normal saline, 25% urethane, 0.1% haparin, 0.01% noradrenaline, 0.1% varapamil, 0.002% dobutamine, 0.0025% cedilanid, 0.5% aminophylline, 1% furosemide.

Experimental subjects

Rabbits weighting about 1.8~2.5 kg.

Experimental procedures

(1) Open the computer and the MedLab A/D converter.

(2) Run the RM6240 EC.

(3) Select "Haemodynamic experiment".

(4) Select "observe".

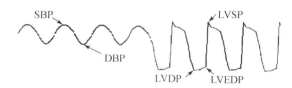

Figure 3-13   Waveform of pressure changes from artery to ventricle.

(5) Select "Observe" and check the signal conduction and keep the signal transmission working.

(6) After weighting the rabbit, it is anaesthetized with urethane injection (1g/ kg, 4 ml/kg, 25% solution, from the marginal vein in the ear). The rabbit is to be placed and fixed by rope on the operating table. After isolating the bilateral carotid artery, use a surgical thread to tie the distal end, and put a surgical thread on the proximal end. Use arterial clamps to block blood flow from the proximal end and make a little incision on the artery, insert a plastic tube (cardiac catheter) of diameter of 2 mm filled with 0.1% heparin solution (ensure that no air bubble in the tube) into the right carotid artery. When inserting the tube into artery, you will see the wave of blood pressure. Then insert the tube forward continuously until the amplitude of wave becomes abruptly larger that means the tube has reached the ventricle.

If the wave of blood pressure disappears, that means the cardiac catheter touched the wall of the vessel. Stop inserting the cardiac tube to avoid transpiercing the artery wall. The tube should be retreated (moved tube backward) till the wave recur and then change a direction to insert the tube Insert an arterial catheter into the left carotid artery for measuring of arterial blood pressure. Select real-time measurement. Record the normal hearmodynamic measurements after stabilization for about 5 min.

(7) Heart failure rabbit model:

The heart failure model could be made by the following

① Inject a large volume of normal saline to the marginal vein in the rabbit's ear rapidly (5~8 ml/kg /min, 5 minutes), while making a "marker" (saline). When the + dp/dt max value obviously declines to half of the normal, heart failure may take place.

② If heart failure does not occur, inject 0.01% noradrenaline (1 ml/kg) to marginal vein in the rabbit ear, then observe the change of hemodynamic parameters to judge whether the heart failure take place. (When the peripheral resistance is increased too much to be overcome by the heart, heart failure will take place.)

③ If heart failure still does not occur, inject 0.1% verapamil (0.2 ml /kg) slowly, then observe the change of hemodynamic parameters to judge occurrence of the heart failure. If verapamil is injected too much, there is no chance to rescue heart failure.

(8) When heart failure occurs, inject 0.0025% Cedilanid (a cardiac glycoside), or 0.002% dobutamine, or 0.5% aminophylline (0.1 ml/kg), or 1% furosemide respectively. Record the changes of hemodynamic parameters for 5 min after each administration.

(9) Name and reserve the experiment data.

(10) Select data and static measurement, edit all data into a clear table, and then print it.

(11) Analyze the data and explain the mechanism of drugs used in this experiment, and write the experimental report.

Table 3-17　Experimental results

Drugs	SP	DP	HR	LVSP	LVDP	$+dp/dt$ max	$-dp/dt$ max	$t-dp/dt$ max
Normal								
Normal saline								
Noradrenaline								
Varapamil								
Dobutamine								
Cedilanid								
Aminophylline								
Furosemide								

Notices

(1) Remember to make a marker before each injection of drug.

(2) After finishing experiment, every group should clean the tables and instruments, and record the results of the experiment.

Questions and discussion

(1) How many heart failure models could be made? Explain the principles.

(2) Why are the drugs (Cedilanid , dobutamine, aminophylline and furosemide) used in treating heart failure?

(3) What are the hemodynamic parameters for evaluation of cardiac function? What are their meanings?

(Xiaodong Wu)

第四章　机能学虚拟实验

一、系统概述

机能学自主学习平台是由南京医科大学主持与东南大学、南京易迪优软件开发有限公司联合开发的网络虚拟自主学习平台。平台从教学目标、教学内容和教学策略进行学习平台构建。医学基础实验对医科学生具有重要意义,医学实验开放因涉及实验动物、实验器械、实验药品及实验教师,需要消耗大量的人力、物力,使得实验开放变得困难,自主学习平台为开放实验提供非常好的辅助手段,为实验开放提供新的解决方案。运用3D技术构建虚拟环境,器材三维展示,其虚拟实验模拟药物及作用因素对呼吸、血压、泌尿的影响曲线;学生利用器材库器材进行实验台的搭建、虚拟手术等;教师可以自定义曲线样式,动态添加实验。机能学自主学习平台包含实验室漫游、动物中心、药品试剂、器械仪器、手术操作、虚拟实验、在线考核等模块,极大地扩展了学生的学习内容与学习空间。

二、系统使用

双击桌面"机能学自主学习平台"快捷方式,启动机能学自主学习平台软件,可见图4-1中各模块,下面对各模块进行简述。

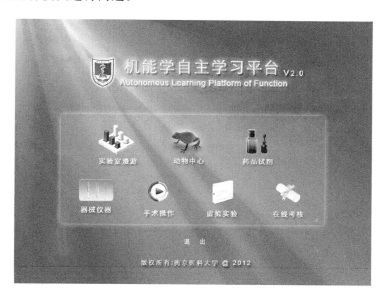

图 4-1　软件主界面图

1. 实验室漫游

运用3DMAX构建实验场景(图4-2),介绍机能实验室房间布置及功能分布,学生可以在三维场景中环绕,并可点击里面的热区进行功能了解。

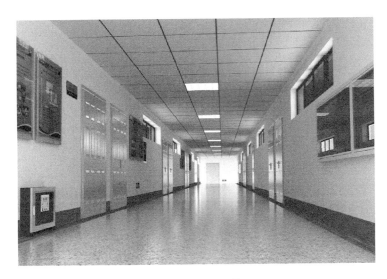

图 4-2　实验区 3D 模拟图

2. 动物中心

动物中心对实验动物的相关知识进行系统全面介绍(图 4-3),动物中心模块下设实验动物、动物选择、性别鉴定、编号与分组、捉持与固定、动物麻醉等结构,鼠标移动到某一个模块上时,相关部分会发光,鼠标点击,在右侧即可显示该部分的缩略图,在图标上点击即可打开学习。在具体学习内容的横排菜单栏的不同菜单上点击,即可进行相关知识学习。

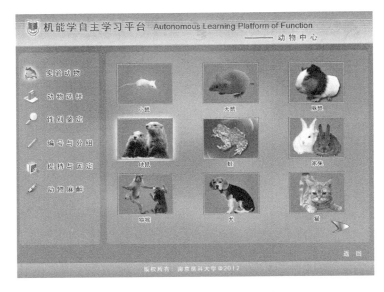

图 4-3　动物中心功能学习平台

3. 药品试剂

药品试剂模块下设实验药物、麻醉药物、单位浓度换算、试剂配制等结构,鼠标移动到某一个模块上时,相关部分会发光,鼠标点击,在右侧即可显示相关结构的内容(图 4-4),在其右侧的图标上点击即可进入相应药物知识的学习。

实验药物
麻醉药物
单位浓度换算
试剂配制
乙醚
混合麻醉剂

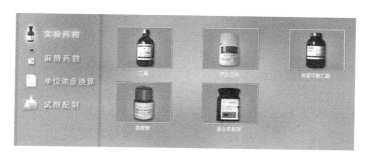

图 4-4　药品试剂模块首页

在各个部分不同的横排菜单(图 4-5)上点击,可以学习该菜单下知识。

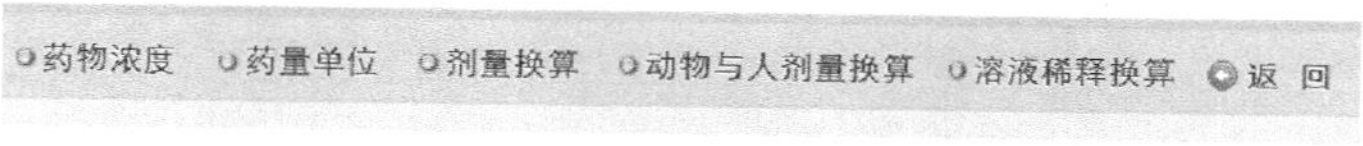

药物浓度
药量单位
剂量换算
动物与人剂量换算
溶液稀释换算
返 回

图 4-5　具体药剂相关内容

4. 器械仪器

当鼠标移动至主页面"器械仪器"或其图标时,其相应图标、文字都会发光,点击即可进入其模块页面,左侧为目录结构(如图 4-6),点击目录树的"+",可以伸展目录下的内容,点击"-",可以收缩其目录下面的内容,在展开后无加减号的文件夹图标上点击,在页面的右侧可以看见在此目录下面的仪器缩略图片。点击缩略图即可在页面的中间看到器材图形,在页面下面可以看到器材的简介(如图 4-7)。点击页面上的"退出",即可回到主页面。

医学器械
01蛙类手术器械
01剪刀
02镊子
03玻璃分针
04金属探针
05锌铜弓
06蛙板
06蛙心夹
02哺乳类手术器械
03基础手术器械
04.实验仪器

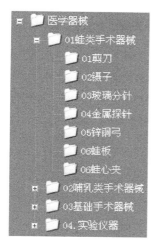

图 4-6

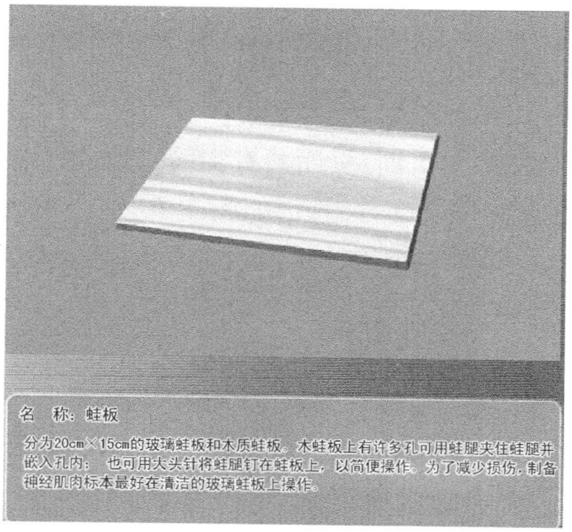

名　称:蛙板
分为20cm×15cm的玻璃蛙板和木质蛙板。木蛙板上有许多孔可用蛙腿夹住蛙腿并嵌入孔内; 也可用大头针将蛙腿钉在蛙板上,以简便操作。为了减少损伤,制备神经肌肉标本最好在清洁的玻璃蛙板上操作。

图 4-7

5. 手术操作

当鼠标移动至主页面"手术操作"或其图标时,其相应图标、文字都会发光,点击即可进入其模块页面,左侧为目录结构(操作方法与图 4-6 相同),点击目录树的"+",可以伸展目录下的内容"-",在目录结构完全伸展开以后就可以看到手术操作过程的视频文件名称,他们前面有一个播放器图标"▶",当我们点击相应手术操作的视频文件名称(或者"▶"图标)

时候,我们即可在右侧播放器中看到我们点击的内容,点击页面上的"退出",即可回到主页面。

6. 虚拟实验

(1)实验项目页面:当鼠标移动至主页面"虚拟实验"或其图标时,其相应图标、文字都会发光,点击即可进入其模块页面。这个模块页面显示是实验分类和实验项目,目前机能学实验分生理、药理、病生(病理生理)和其他等模块组成(如图4-8)。点击图4-8中某项分类,右侧即可出现该分类下的实验项目(如图4-9),当鼠标移到某个实验项目上时候,其图标就会发光,点击即可进入仿真实验界面,如果实验项目中有下一页图标(如图4-10),表示有多页面,点击即可看到下一个页面的实验项目,在页面中有上一页图标(如图4-11),点击即可回到上一个项目页面。点击"退出"即可退到客户端主页面。

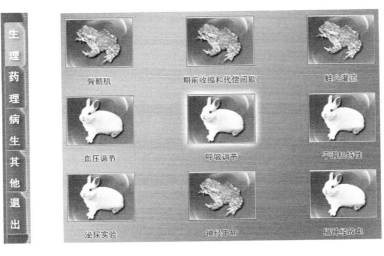

图 4-8 　　　　　　　　　　　　　　　　图 4-9 　　　　　　　　　　图 4-10 　　图 4-11

(2)虚拟实验主页面:页面共有实验步骤、虚拟操作、实验对象、仿真实战、实验试剂、实验器材、实验简介等7部分组成(如图4-12)。当我们鼠标移动到相应模块上时,会有相应

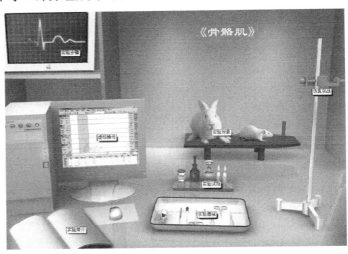

图 4-12　仿真实验主页面

118

模块名称的提示出现，点击即可显示该部分内容，点击关闭按钮“×”即可关闭相应显示内容。但是需要注意：点击“虚拟实验”会进入药物及处理的波形仿真的新页面；点击“虚拟操作”时候如果该实验没有相应内容会跳出对话框提示用户，如果有则会进入相应的新页面中。

(3) “虚拟实验”页面：页面有波形显示区用于显示动物的呼吸、血压、谜尿、标记等信息(如图 4-13)；在波形显示区右侧有一排快捷工具栏，用于对波形进行设置(如图 4-14)；作用因素用于放置实验各种药物以及处理因素，点击作用处理图标即可对动物进行作用(如图 4-15)，此时会对动物的呼吸、血压、谜尿、标记等信息引起变化，反映在波形显示区内；药物浓度区是表现在给了作用因素(刺激、处理、药物等)后其效果在动物体内的变化情况(如图 4-16)；波形控制区就是对各种波形进行控制(如图 4-17)；动物反映区表现出在给过各种作用处理后，动物的变化情况。

400
200
0
−200
−400

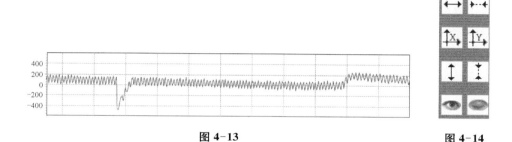

图 4-13

图 4-14

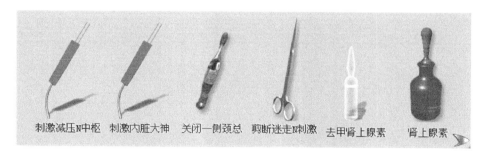

刺激减压N中枢
刺激内脏大神
关闭一侧颈总
剪断迷走N刺激
去甲肾上腺素
肾上腺素

图 4-15

药量浓度
去甲肾上腺素

图 4-16

波形控制
暂停
快速
换洗
退出

图 4-17

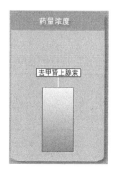

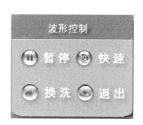

（4）功能说明：①图 4-14 功能说明：↔对波形进行横向拉伸；↦对波形进行横向压缩；↤使波形横向还原到初始状态；↕对波形进行纵向拉伸；↨对波形进行纵向压缩；↥使波形纵向还原到初始状态；●关闭波形中的尺度显示；●打开波形中的尺度显示。②图 4-17 功能说明：[Ⅱ 暂停]对波形进行暂停继续等处理；[◎ 快速]加速波形的移动速度；[● 换洗]取消动物的处理作用还原到正常的初始状态；[● 退出]退出当前页面回到仿真实验主页面。

7. 在线考核

当鼠标移动至主页面"在线考核"或其图标时，其相应图标、文字都会发光，点击即可进入其模块页面，它分生理学、药理学、病理生理学、生物化学、综合试题。点击相应部分左侧就会显示它相应的章节目录，点击章节，在左侧题目显示区就会显示该章节包含的题目，当您做完题目后，在题目的最下面有一个答案提交按钮，提交就可以对您的答题作一个测评，系统会显示您哪些题目正确，哪些答错，对于答错的会给出相应题目正确答案，最后会给出一个本章自测的正确率，点击页面上的"退出"，即可回到主页面。

药物考核主要考核多种药物之间的相互影响，其使用与"虚拟实验"中使用一致，可以参考"虚拟实验"中（3）与（4）。

三、退出客户端系统

点击主页面上的"退出"，进入退出页面，在退出页面的文字上单击即可退出当前客户端。

（袁艺标）

第五章　机能实验学综合实验设计

"机能实验学综合实验设计"课程是以活体动物为实验对象,实施以教师为主导,学生为主体的研究性学习,培养学生创新意识,开拓学生科研思维,提升临床技能素质的重要实践平台。

进行机能实验学综合实验设计是实施研究性学习的关键环节。所设计的实验是建立在科学基础之上,除要具备一定的基础知识外,还应具有一定的观察、发现问题的能力和一定的创造能力。理解和掌握实验设计的基本知识对于提高教学质量,推进以创新教育为核心的素质教育有重要作用,设计实验方案是培养综合能力中较高层次的要求,亦是科学素养的重要组成部分。

综合实验设计教学程序分三方面进行:课堂讲授有关实验设计与实验研究的基本内容;学生自行查阅相关文献资料;学生在预实验中修改、完善实验设计,体验了解科研过程与科研思维。实施研讨型学习模式,达到培养学生创新能力,提高其科学素质的教学目的。

一、综合实验设计的设计原则

(一)科研设计的三大原则:

1. 对照原则

在实验研究中需设对照组或对照试验。其目的在于鉴别干预因素与非干预因素之间的差异。以消除和减少实验误差。对照应符合均衡原则。在相互比较的各组之间(实验组与对照组之间、实验组与实验组之间)除了要研究的干预因素有差别之外,其他一切条件。如动物的数量、种系、性别、重量、实验方法、仪器、药品、环境等均应力求一致。

(1)空白对照:对照组不加任何处理因素。

(2)自身对照:同一个动物上先后给予两次处理,如先用生理盐水,后用某种干预用的药品。

(3)组间对照:几个实验组之间相互对照(包括阳性对照组)。

2. 随机原则:

随机的方法有随机数目表、抽签法。其目的是:

(1)是每一个样本在实验中有同等的机会,尽量使抽取的样本能代表总体,减少抽样误差。

(2)使各组样本的条件尽量一致,消除或减少实验者因主观原因产生的误差,从而使干预因素产生的作用更加客观。

3. 重复原则

由于实验动物存在个体差异与实验误差的影响,仅在一个样本或一次实验得到的结果不够切实可信,必须要有一定的重复,才能保证结果的可靠性。在设计中,对样本大小的估计原则是保证确切科学的基础上用最少的数目。一般而言,计数指标每组不应少于30列,计量指标每组不能少于6列。

(二)疾病动物模型的设计原则

在机能实验学综合实验设计中,往往要探索一些重大疾病的发生发展规律与机制,需要设计制备疾病动物模型。

1. 设计模型需要注意的原则

(1)相似性:复制的疾病动物模型应尽可能近似于人类疾病。

(2)重复性:疾病动物模型是可重复和可标准化的。

(3)可靠性:复制的疾病动物模型应具有该疾病的症状与体征,能可靠地反映该疾病的代谢与结构的变化。

(4)经济性:制备模型的方法简单易行,经济实惠,便于观察。

2. 综合实验设计的立题

进行综合实验设计首先要确定一个实验研究的课题,在学生现有医学基本理论与实践的基础上,提出一个需探索研究的问题或设想。而后让学生充分查阅文献,了解该问题产生的背景,形成一个确切的科学假设。将假设进一步概括即形成实验设计的题目。

一个优秀的实验设计题目应具有:

(1)科学性:所立题目应有充分的科学依据,与已有的科学理论与科学规律相符。

(2)目的性:明确所要研究的问题,提出具体的解决方案。

(3)创新性:通过查阅大量的文献,尽量避免重复前人的实验。实验研究必须要有新意,要有探索创新的亮点。

(4)可行性:立题时要考虑实验方面相关的主客观条件,从实际出发,在条件许可范围内进行立题。

立题范围也可参考以下几个方面:

(1)改进原有的实验教学方法,对其进行深入或拓展。

(2)建立某疾病或病理过程的实验动物模型并评价该模型的指标

(3)验证一种假说

(4)探索某因素在某种疾病发生发展中的作用

(5)揭示某疾病或病理过程新的机能代谢变化及其机制

(6)探讨对某疾病或病理过程的药物治疗方法

二、机能实验学综合实验设计的具体内容

1. 综合实验设计的题目

2. 立题依据

主要阐述你"为什么"要研究设计这个题目?

(1)阐述研究背景:围绕着设计题目所提出的假设,阐述国内外目前对该领域的研究概况;

(2)提出研究目的与研究意义:在阐述、分析研究概况的基础上,引出你研究该内容的目的及意义。

立题依据的书写要在充分查阅文献资料的基础上进行,围绕着研究假设,充分体现该研究设计的科学性与创新性。

3. 研究内容与研究方法(技术路线)

具体说明你将"怎么做"做这个题目

提出完成这个实验研究的具体实施方案。其包括:

(1)依据研究的内容与目的,选择实验动物并设置相应的分组(如对照组)。要写明动物的名称、品种、性别、体重、健康状况。

(2)依据研究的内容与目的,按研究的层次与水平,选择相应的实验方法与观测指标。要注重各种方法的互相补充,互相印证而获得可信的结果。既要有科学性、先进性;又要有可行性。观测指标亦要体现其灵敏性、重现性、特异性。

(3)设计研究试验中的干预处理因素,并要评估其作用效应。

(4)确定适当的统计方法。

(5)实验中的实验器材和药品:主要仪器的名称、型号、厂家,药品的名称、厂家,试剂的浓度,剂量,给药的途径。

(6)若设计中需要制备疾病动物模型,则要详细说明模型制备的方法与判断造模成功的标准。

4. 实验设计中要有预实验结果

科学合理的实验设计并非是一次性就能完成。在实验正式开始之前,一定先要做预实验。预实验是根据综合设计要求,通过几组非正式的简单实验对其设计的"原始假说"进行初步验证,或对实验中将要出现的技术难点或关键性指标进行出版的实验观察,以判断实验设计的可行性。

通过预实验熟悉实验设计中所需的方法与技术,亦有利于严谨、细致、全面系统地观察实验结果,并要及时做好原始的实验记录。可预先设计好实验结果的原始记录方式,这一点非常重要。因为它是整个实验的结晶,是实验全过程的最终收获!

设计者可根据预实验的结果,对综合实验设计做进一步的修改。

(董榕)

附录一　常用药物及试剂

表1　常用生理溶液的成分和含量

试剂及剂量	台式液用于哺乳类（小肠）	乐氏液用于两栖类	任氏液用于两栖类	生理盐水	
				两栖类	哺乳类
NaCl（g）	8.00	9.00	6.50	6.50	9.00
KCl（g）	0.20	0.42	0.14	—	—
CaCl₂（g）	0.20	0.24	0.12	—	—
NaHCO₃（g）	1.00	0.10～0.30	0.20	—	—
NaH₂PO₄（g）	0.05	—	0.01	—	—
MgCl₂（g）	0.10	—	—	—	—
Glucose（g）	1.00	1.00～2.50	2.00(可不加)	—	—
蒸馏水加至(ml)	1 000	1 000	1 000	1 000	1 000

表2　人和动物间按体表面积折算的等效剂量比率表

		小白鼠 20 g	大白鼠 200 g	豚鼠 400 g	兔 1.5 kg	猫 2.0 kg	猴 4.0 kg	狗 12.0 kg	人 70.0 kg
小白鼠	20 g	1.000 0	7.000	12.250	27.80	29.700	64.10	124.20	387.9
大白鼠	200 g	0.140 0	1.000	1.240	3.90	4.200	9.20	17.80	56.0
豚鼠	400 g	0.800 0	0.570	1.000	2.25	2.400	5.20	4.20	31.5
兔	1.5 kg	0.040 0	0.250	0.440	1.00	1.080	2.40	4.50	41.2
猫	2.0 kg	0.030 0	0.230	0.410	0.92	1.000	2.20	4.10	31.0
猴	4.0 kg	0.016 0	0.110	0.190	0.42	0.450	1.00	1.90	6.1
狗	12.0 kg	0.008 0	0.060	0.100	0.22	0.230	0.52	1.00	3.1
人	70.0 kg	0.002 6	0.018	0.031	0.07	0.078	0.16	0.32	1.0

表3　非挥发性麻醉药的用法和用量

药物	动物	给药途径	剂量(mg/kg)	麻醉时间和特点
戊巴比妥钠（3%～5%）	狗、兔	静脉注射	25～30	2～4h,中途补充5 mg/kg可维持1 h以上。对呼吸血压影响较小,肌肉松弛不全,麻醉稳定。常用。
	猫	腹腔注射	30	
	豚鼠、大白鼠、小白鼠	腹腔注射	40～50	

药物	动物	给药途径	剂量(mg/kg)	麻醉时间和特点
异戊巴比妥钠(5%)	兔	静脉注射	40～50	约2～4h,对呼吸血压影响较小,肌肉松弛不全,麻醉不稳定。
	鼠	腹腔注射	80～1000	
硫喷妥钠(5%)	狗、兔	静脉注射	20～30	约0.5h静注宜缓以抑制呼吸致死,肌肉松弛不全。
	猫	腹腔注射	30～50	
乌拉坦(25%)	兔、猫	静注、腹腔注射、灌胃	1 000～1 450	2～4h,麻醉较好,可用于生理神经发射性实验。
	鼠	腹腔注射	1 000～1 500	
氯醛糖(2%)	狗	静脉注射	80～100	6h,可用于生理神经反射性实验。
氯醛糖+乌拉坦	狗	静脉注射	氯 50～60 乌 500～600	
	猫	静脉注射	氯 60 乌 800	
	豚鼠	腹腔注射	氯 20 乌 1000	
苯巴比妥钠(20%)	狗	静脉注射	30～100	8h,对呼吸血压影响较小,肌肉松弛不全。少用。
	猫、兔、鼠	静脉或腹腔注射	80～100	
巴比妥钠(10%)	狗	静脉注射	250～300	同上
	猫、兔、鼠	静脉或腹腔注射	200	

表4 常用血液抗凝剂

抗凝剂	用法
枸橼酸钠	常用3.8%的溶液。一般以血液9份,加此液1份。因其抗凝作用较弱,且碱性较强,不宜作化学检验之用。可用于红细胞沉降速度测定。急性血压实验所用的枸橼酸钠为5%～7%溶液。
草酸钾	用10%草酸钾溶液,吸取0.2 ml于一试管内,旋转试管,使溶液浸润试管,然后放在烘箱中(80℃)烤干、包好备用。每支如此制备的试管、可使10 ml血不凝。如加血量不到10 ml,可按比例减少草酸钾溶液量,草酸钾过多可引起溶血。
肝素	市售肝素溶液每ml含肝素12 500国际单位,相当于125 mg(即1 mg相当于100 U)。 体外抗凝:取肝素溶液0.1 ml于试管内,均匀湿润后,放入烘箱(80～100℃)烤干,每管能使10ml血不凝。 体内抗凝:静脉注射500～1000 U/kg。

抗凝剂	用　　法
草酸钾-草酸铵混合剂	草酸钾 0.8 g、草酸铵 1.2 g 加蒸馏水至 100 ml，取 0.5 ml 置于试管内，烘干备用。每管能使 10 ml 血不凝。此抗凝剂适于作红细胞比容测定，但不能用于血液非蛋白氮测定。

附录二　病　案　讨　论

一、目的

运用学过的病理生理学等知识对临床病例进行分析,作出初步诊断,并提出诊断依据、主要疾病的发展过程及相关临床表现的病理机制,以巩固所学的病理生理学理论基础知识。

二、病历摘要

患者宋××,男,68岁,农民。因反复咳嗽、咯痰22年,心悸、气急、水肿2年,加重半月,于2012年12月13日14:30急诊入院。

患者自1990年起,每遇天气转冷,咳嗽、咯痰即发作,清晨咳嗽较剧、痰量少,多为白色黏痰。无气急、气喘、咯血及盗汗。每次发作持续7~10天,经青霉素、咳喘宁等药治疗,即可好转,每年发作2~3次,多在秋末冬初时。工作、生活不受影响。2002年以来,咳嗽、咯痰加重,早晚尤剧,有时伴气短。每日痰量10~20 ml,为白色泡沫样,需青霉素等药物治疗方可缓解。每次持续3个月以上,天气转暖时上述症状缓解。干重活则有心悸、气急感,但日常生活尚可自理。2010年冬起,咳嗽及咯白色泡沫痰终年不断,无明显季节性。常有发热,多在38℃左右。痰量每日50~60 ml,发热时痰量可增至100 ml左右,呈黄色脓性痰、伴气急、心悸、双下肢浮肿。动则气急、心悸加重。日常生活不能完全自理,有时静卧亦觉气急。

此次于11月28日受凉后又发病,咯黄色脓性痰、不易咯出。心悸、气急加重,双下肢浮肿,尿量减少,口唇发绀。进食少许即觉上腹部饱胀不适,并有轻度恶心。经青霉素、头孢菌素、沐舒坦、氢氯噻嗪等药治疗未见好转,于今日送我院急诊。

平素身体较差,幼年曾患"麻疹、水痘、流腮"等传染病。2006年经X线钡餐摄片检查诊断为"胃下垂"。2008年因尿潴留诊断为"前列腺肥大",目前尚有排尿困难、夜间尿频。

吸烟40年,每天10支左右,2002年已戒烟。否认家族中有传染病及遗传病史。

1. 体格检查

体温36.1℃,脉搏104次/min,呼吸32次/min,血压12.0/8.0 kPa(90/60 mmHg),发育正常。营养中等,慢性重病容,神志清楚。取半坐卧位,呼吸及语言困难,烦躁,体检欠合作。未见巩膜及皮肤黄染,未见浅表淋巴结肿大,未见头颅异常,未见眼睑浮肿。两侧瞳孔等大同圆,对光反应灵敏。耳无脓性分泌物,鼻通气良好,口腔无特殊气味。唇发绀,伸舌居中,咽部充血,未见扁桃体肿大,颈静脉怒张。桶状胸,肋间隙增宽。两侧呼吸运动对称,节律规则,未触及胸膜摩擦感及握雪感。叩诊两肺反响增强,呈过清音。两肺呼吸音较弱,呼气音延长,两肺上部可闻及干性罗音,两肩胛下区可闻细湿罗音。心前区未见隆起,剑突下可见搏动,范围较弥散,未触及震颤。心界叩不出,心率104次/min,心律齐,各瓣音区未闻及病理性杂音,$P_2 > A_2$。腹平软。肝肋缘下3cm,剑突下5 cm,质中,边缘钝,轻度触痛,肝颈静脉回流征(+);脾未触及。全腹未触及包块,未见压痛及反跳痛,未见移动性浊音,肠鸣音正常。未见肛门、外生殖器异常。直肠指诊:前列腺Ⅱ°肥大,质中,表面光滑,中央沟消失。未见运动障碍;未见脊柱、四肢畸形,未见关节红肿、杵状指/趾;双下肢小腿以下呈凹陷性浮肿。腱反射正常,巴宾斯基征阴性。

2. 检验及其他检查

(1)血象:红细胞计数 $4.8 \times 10^{12}/L$(480 万/μL),血红蛋白 156g/L,白细胞计数 $11 \times 10^9/L$ (11 000/μL),中性 80%,淋巴 15%,单核 2%,嗜酸 2%,嗜碱 1% 。

(2)血气分析:pH 7.31,Pa O_2 6.7 kPa(52.5 mmHg),Pa CO_2 8.6 kPa(64.8 mmHg),BE-2.8 mmol/L。

(3)胸部 X 片:两肺透亮度增加,纹理增多、紊乱,肋间隙增宽,右肺下动脉干横径 18 mm。心影大小正常。

(4)心电图:肺性 P 波,电轴右偏,右室肥大。

三、讨论内容

(1)试提出初步诊断。
(2)试说明患者主要疾病与病理过程的发展过程。
(3)从病理生理学角度分析患者的一些临床表现和检验结果。

附:部分临床检验正常参考值(成年男性)

(1)血常规部分项目:红细胞计数 $4.2 \sim 5.4 \times 10^{12}/L$,血红蛋白 120 ~ 160g/L;白细胞计数 $4.0 \sim 10.0 \times 10^9/L$,中性 54%~ 62%,淋巴 25%~ 33%,单核 3%~ 7%,嗜酸 1%~ 4%,嗜碱 0%~ 1%。

(2)血气分析:pH7.35 ~ 7.45,Pa O_2 9.3 ~ 13.3 kPa (70 ~100 mmHg),Pa CO_2 4.5 ~ 6.0KPa (34 ~ 45 mmHg),BE:±3 mmol/L。

(3)胸部 X 片:右肺下动脉干横径<15 mmol。

(余卫平)

参考文献

［1］高兴亚,汪晖,戚晓红,等.机能实验学.北京:科学出版社,2007
［2］陆源,夏强.生理科学实验教程.杭州:浙江大学出版社,2004
［3］郑倩.医学机能学实验.北京:科学出版社,2013
［4］徐叔云,卞如濂,陈修.药理学实验方法.北京:人民卫生出版社,2002
［5］杨芳炬.机能学实验.北京:高等教育出版社,2010
［6］朱大年,王庭槐.生理学.北京:人民卫生出版社,2013
［7］姚泰.生理学.北京:人民卫生出版社,2003
［8］胡还忠.医学机能学实验教程.北京:科学出版社,2010
［9］丁全福.药理实验教程.北京:人民卫生出版社,1996
［10］杨宝峰.药理学.北京:人民卫生出版社,2013
［11］胡维诚.医学机能学实验.北京:科学出版社,2010
［12］袁秉祥,阎剑群.机能实验学.北京:高等教育出版社,2007
［13］娄建石,徐淑梅,刘欣.机能学实验.北京:人民卫生出版社,2007
［14］陈奇.中药药理学研究方法学.北京:人民卫生出版社,2000
［15］方厚华.医学实验模型动物.北京:军事医学科学出版社,2003
［16］郑铁生.临床生物化学检验.北京:中国医药科技出版社,2004
［17］王建枝.病理生理学.北京:人民卫生出版社,2013
［18］郭继军.医学文献检索与论文写作.北京:人民卫生出版社,2013
［19］秦川.医学实验动物学.北京:人民卫生出版社,2008